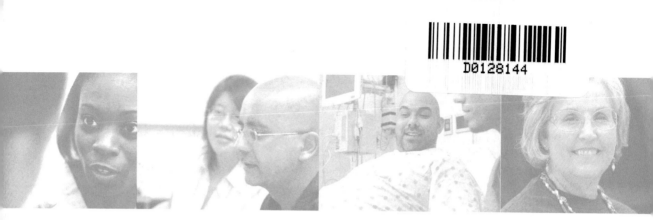

Johns Hopkins Nursing
Evidence-Based Practice
Model and Guidelines

Books Published by the Honor Society of Nursing, Sigma Theta Tau International

Johns Hopkins Nursing Evidence-Based Practice Model and Guidelines, Robin Newhouse, Sandra Dearholt, Stephanie Poe, Linda Pugh, and Kathleen White, 2007.

Nursing Without Borders: Values, Wisdom, Success Markers, Sharon Weinstein and Ann Marie T. Brooks, 2007.

Synergy: The Unique Relationship Between Nurses and Patients, Martha A.Q. Curley, 2007.

Conversations With Leaders: Frank Talk From Nurses (and Others) on the Front Lines of Leadership, Tine Hansen-Turton, Susan Sherman, Vernice Ferguson, 2007.

Pivotal Moments in Nursing: Leaders Who Changed the Path of a Profession, Beth Houser and Kathy Player, 2004 (Volume I) and 2007 (Volume II).

Shared Legacy, Shared Vision: The W. K. Kellogg Foundation and the Nursing Profession, Joan E. Lynaugh, Helen Grace, Gloria R. Smith, Roseni Sena, María Mercedes Durán de Villalobos, and Mary Malehloka Hlalele, 2007.

Daily Miracles: Stories and Practices of Humanity and Excellence in Health Care, Alan Briskin and Jan Boller, 2006.

A Daybook for Nurse Leaders and Mentors, Sigma Theta Tau International, 2006.

When Parents Say No: Religious and Cultural Influences on Pediatric Healthcare Treatment, Luanne Linnard-Palmer, 2006.

Healthy Places, Healthy People: A Handbook for Culturally Competent Community Nursing Practice, Melanie C. Dreher, Dolores Shapiro, and Micheline Asselin, 2006.

The HeART of Nursing: Expressions of Creative Art in Nursing, Second Edition, M. Cecilia Wendler, 2005.

Reflecting on 30 Years of Nursing Leadership: 1975-2005, Sr. Rosemary Donley, 2005

Technological Competency as Caring in Nursing, Rozzano Locsin, 2005.

Making a Difference: Stories from the Point of Care, Volume I1, Sharon Hudacek, 2005.

A Daybook for Nurses: Making a Difference Each Day, Sharon Hudacek, 2004.

Making a Difference: Stories from the Point of Care, Volume II, Sharon Hudacek, 2004.

Building and Managing a Career in Nursing: Strategies for Advancing Your Career, Terry Miller, 2003.

Collaboration for the Promotion of Nursing, LeAlice Briggs, Sonna Ehrlich Merk, and Barbara Mitchell, 2003.

Ordinary People, Extraordinary Lives: The Stories of Nurses, Carolyn Smeltzer and Frances Vlasses, 2003.

Stories of Family Caregiving: Reconsideration of Theory, Literature, and Life, Suzanne Poirier and Lioness Ayres, 2002.

As We See Ourselves: Jewish Women in Nursing, Evelyn Benson, 2001.

Cadet Nurse Stories: The Call for and Response of Women During World War II, Thelma Robinson and Paulie Perry, 2001.

Creating Responsive Solutions to Healthcare Change, Cynthia McCullough, 2001.

The Language of Nursing Theory and Metatheory, Imogene King and Jacqueline Fawcett, 1997.

nurseAdvance Collection. (Topic-specific collections of honor society published journal articles.) Topics are: Cardiovascular Nursing; Cultural Diversity in Nursing; Disaster, Trauma, and Emergency Nursing; Ethical and Legal Issues in Nursing; Genomics in Nursing and Healthcare; Gerontological Nursing; Health Promotion in Nursing; Implementing Evidence-Based Nursing; Leadership and Mentoring in Nursing; Maternal Health Nursing; Oncology Nursing; Pain Management in Nursing; Pediatric Nursing; Psychiatric-Mental Health Nursing; Public, Environmental, and Community Health Nursing; and Women's Health Nursing; 2007.

To order any of these books, visit Nursing Knowledge International's website at **www.nursingknowledge.org/stti/books**. Nursing Knowledge International is the honor society's sales and distribution division. You may also call 1.888.NKI.4.YOU (U.S. and Canada) or +1.317.634.8171 (Outside U.S. and Canada) to place an order.

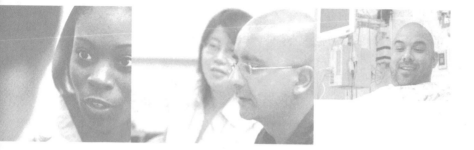
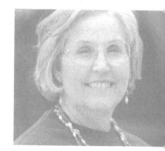

Johns Hopkins Nursing
Evidence-Based Practice
Model and Guidelines

Robin P. Newhouse, PhD, RN, CNA, CNOR
Sandra L. Dearholt, MS, RN
Stephanie S. Poe, MScN, RN
Linda C. Pugh, PhD, RNC, FAAN
Kathleen M. White, PhD, RN, CNAA, BC

Sigma Theta Tau International
Honor Society of Nursing®

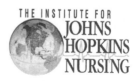

THE INSTITUTE FOR
JOHNS
HOPKINS
NURSING

Sigma Theta Tau International

Editor-in-Chief: Jeff Burnham
Acquisitions Editor: Cynthia L. Saver, RN, MS
Project Editor: Carla Hall
Development and Copy Editor: Brian Walls
Editorial Team: Melody Jones, Jane Palmer
Indexer: Julie Bess

Cover Design: Gary Adair
Interior Design and Page Composition: Rebecca Harmon

Printed in the United States of America
Printing and Binding by Printing Partners, Indianapolis, Indiana, USA

Sigma Theta Tau International
550 West North Street
Indianapolis, IN 46202

Visit our Web site at www.nursingknowledge.org/STTI/books for more information on our books.
ISBN-13: 978-1-930538-71-9
ISBN-10: 1-930538-71-5

Library of Congress Cataloging-in-Publication Data

The Johns Hopkins nursing evidence-based practice model and guidelines / Robin P. Newhouse ... [et al.].

     p. ; cm.

Includes bibliographical references.

ISBN-13: 978-1-930538-71-9

ISBN-10: 1-930538-71-5

1. Evidence-based nursing. 2. Nursing models. I. Newhouse, Robin Purdy. II. Sigma Theta Tau International. III. Johns Hopkins Hospital. IV. Johns Hopkins University. School of Nursing. V. Title: Nursing evidence-based practice model and guidelines.

[DNLM: 1. Nursing Process. 2. Evidence-Based Medicine. 3. Models, Nursing. WY 100 J65 2007]

RT42.J62 2007

610.73—dc22

                              2007040291

Second Printing 2008

DEDICATION

This book is dedicated to the advancement of evidence-based practice (EBP) as a critical competency for all nurses.

ACKNOWLEDGEMENTS

The authors would like to acknowledge Karen Haller, PhD, RN, FAAN, Martha Hill, PhD, RN, FAAN, and Deborah Dang, PhD, RN, for their visionary leadership and support for weaving evidence-based practice into the fabric of Johns Hopkins Nursing.

ABOUT THE AUTHORS

Robin P. Newhouse, PhD, RN, CNA, CNOR

At the time this book was written, Dr. Newhouse was nurse researcher at The Johns Hopkins Hospital and assistant professor at The Johns Hopkins University School of Nursing, where she was dedicated to building evidence-based practice and research infrastructure and teaching Application of Research to Practice in the graduate program. She is now associate professor and assistant dean, Doctor of Nursing Practice Program at the University of Maryland, Baltimore School of Nursing, where she continues her work in building nurse leaders with strong evidence-based practice skills. She has published and presented widely on the topic of evidence-based practice and is an active health services researcher who studies organizational and nursing processes and related outcomes. Dr. Newhouse and the co-authors of this book led the development and evaluation of The Johns Hopkins Nursing Evidence-Based Practice Model. This model was highlighted by the Health Care Advisory Board as a best practice in 2005 and won the 2005 International Research Utilization Award from the Honor Society of Nursing, Sigma Theta Tau International.

Sandra L. Dearholt, MS, RN

Ms. Sandra L. Dearholt is the assistant director of nursing for the departments of neuroscience and psychiatry at The Johns Hopkins Hospital. She is a member of The Johns Hopkins Nursing Evidence-Based Practice (JHNEBP) steering committee that developed and implemented the JHNEBP Model. Ms. Dearholt has an extensive background in the development of nursing standards of practice and care and has served in the capacity of coordinator of nursing practice for John Hopkins Nursing. She is currently a member of the Maryland Board of Nursing Practice Issues Committee. Ms. Dearholt is committed to teaching and developing the evidence-based practice and critical thinking skills of the bedside clinician. She has presented the concepts of evidence-based practice in a variety of venues and has co-authored several articles on nursing and evidence-based practice.

Stephanie S. Poe, MScN, RN

Ms. Poe is assistant director of nursing, clinical quality at The Johns Hopkins Hospital and holds a joint appointment with The Johns Hopkins University School of Nursing. She has extensive experience working with nurse leaders and bedside nurses in developing and monitoring care standards to maintain high quality, safe patient care. Ms. Poe helped develop the Johns Hopkins Nursing Evidence-Based Practice Model and has taught and mentored project teams using the model and guidelines. She has published and presented on the topics of evidence-based practice, quality improvement, and patient safety. Ms. Poe's area of research focus is quality improvement, risk assessment, and application of clinical practice guidelines.

Linda C. Pugh, PhD, RNC, FAAN

Dr. Linda C. Pugh is a professor of nursing at York College of Pennsylvania in York, Pennsylvania. She is also the director of EBP/nursing research at York Hospital. Dr. Pugh is the former director of the baccalaureate program at the Johns Hopkins University School of Nursing in Baltimore, Maryland. She has been an active part of the development and implementation of the JHNEBP Model, leading clinicians in advancing their practice through EBP projects. As a certified obstetric nurse, she has provided care for childbearing women for more than 30 years. The focus of her research is improving breastfeeding outcomes, particularly those of low-income women. Dr. Pugh has researched strategies to increase the exclusivity and duration of breastfeeding. She has published and presented her work internationally and nationally. She is also a fellow in the American Academy of Nursing.

Kathleen M. White, PhD, RN, CNAA, BC

Kathleen M. White, PhD, RN, CNAA, BC, is an asociate professor and director for the master's program at The Johns Hopkins University School of Nursing. She holds a joint appointment as clinical nurse specialist at The Johns Hopkins Hospital and nurse research liaison at Howard County General Hospital. She is a member of the team that developed the Johns Hopkins Nursing Evidence-Based Practice Model and guidelines and has consulted locally and nationally about the model. Dr. White has been an active participant in several quality and safety initiatives and has received numerous practice grants. She is a member of the Maryland Health Care Commission's Hospital Performance Evaluation Guide Advisory Committee, a member of the board of directors of Carefirst Blue Cross and Blue Shield and its mission oversight and strategic planning sub-committees, and the interim chairperson of the Maryland Patient Safety Center's board of directors.

TABLE OF CONTENTS

FOREWORD

It is our pleasure to bring you *Johns Hopkins Nursing Evidence-Based Practice Model and Guidelines*, created and tested by a team of nurses and faculty at The Johns Hopkins Hospital and The Johns Hopkins University School of Nursing. Evidence-based practice is important to the safety of our patients, the development of our profession, and the education of our students. It is increasingly the foundation for policies and procedures in health-care settings and the curriculum at many schools of nursing. We believe every nurse needs to understand and use the principles of evidence-based practice to make critical patient-care decisions. This book describes a rigorous, but user-friendly, approach to the challenge of implementing evidence-based practice.

Extensively used by nurses, multidisciplinary teams, faculty, and students, the Johns Hopkins Nursing Evidence-Based Practice Model (JHNEBP) makes evidence-based practice achievable. As you read this book, you will discover guidelines and tools that accompany the description of the model and examples of its application. Our authors take an orderly approach, offering strategies for success at each step in the EBP process. Their goal is to supply nurses with the basic knowledge and skills needed to participate in, and lead, evidence-based practice projects.

After testing the JHNEBP in our organizations, we adopted it as the standard for developing nursing practice recommendations at The Johns Hopkins Hospital. Our baccalaureate and graduate classrooms use the JHNEBP to teach evidence-based practice and develop critical thinking skills. We also shared the JHNEBP with other academic medical centers and with community and rural hospitals. Our authors consulted with those organizations to provide immersion workshops that stepped project teams through a successful evidence-based practice project. This book includes the lessons learned from these applications of the JHNEBP model. Additionally, the authors have tested and refined its components and enhanced their descriptions of its use.

Johns Hopkins Nursing Evidence-Based Practice Model and Guidelines provides background on evidence-based practice, examples of successful EBP projects, and step-by-step guidelines for planning and developing an EBP program—all the tools, tips, and resources required to participate in and conduct evidence-based practice projects. We are proud to offer this contribution to nursing practice and science, and we hope that you will use it to improve your nursing care.

Martha N. Hill, PhD, RN, FAAN
Dean, The Johns Hopkins University School of Nursing

Karen Haller, PhD, RN, FAAN
Vice President for Nursing and Patient Care Services
The Johns Hopkins Hospital

Introduction

Johns Hopkins Nursing Evidence-Based Practice Model and Guidelines is dedicated to the advancement of evidence-based practice (EBP)—a new competency for nurses. The goal of EBP is to promote effective nursing interventions, efficient care, and improved outcomes for patients, and to provide the best available evidence for clinical, administrative, and educational decision making. In today's complex and dynamic patient-care environment, nursing interventions and processes informed by the best evidence are vital to realizing health-care improvements and cost savings. The six sections of this book provide nurses with the critical knowledge, skills, and abilities required to lead evidence-based initiatives in any health-care environment.

Section I introduces the EBP concept. Chapter 1 discusses background information, provides a definition of EBP, and describes the evolution of EBP within the nursing profession. Chapter 2 centers on the role of critical thinking in EBP, its relationship to the nursing process, and its significance in developing practice questions, appraising evidence, and translating findings in the practice setting.

Section II is an overview of the Johns Hopkins Nursing Evidence-Based Practice Model (JHNEBP). Chapter 3 introduces the JHNEBP Model, which frames research and non-research evidence within a professional nursing environment that emphasizes practice, education, and research. Section II closes with guidelines for conducting an EBP project using the Practice question, Evidence, and Translation process (PET).

Section III focuses on the PET process and provides guidance on facilitating project work. Chapter 4 illuminates the practice question by exploring the origin of EBP questions, the criteria for project selection, and the development of an answerable EBP question. Chapters 5, 6, and 7 discuss evidence. Chapter 5 reviews evidence search strategies, online and Web resources, and tips for performing evidence searches. Chapter 6 discusses research evidence, the appraisal process, and appraising and grading evidence. Chapter 7 frames non-research evidence within the PET process. Chapter 8 describes translation, which defines the criteria needed to make an evidence-based practice decision, and includes creating an action plan, making the change, and sharing the findings.

In Section IV, Chapter 9 outlines the environment needed for nurses to incorporate EBP. Lessons in leadership to create and sustain a supportive practice setting and strategies for encouraging and mentoring staff are included.

Section V provides exemplars of projects at The Johns Hopkins Hospital and two community hospitals that illustrate application of the JHNEBP Model and PET process.

Section VI, the Appendixes, includes the JHNEBP Model, a figure of the PET process, and tools for project management, question development, evidence appraisal, rating scales, and individual and overall summaries. These tools are regularly reviewed and updated by the JHNEBP Steering Committee. The reader may download the most current versions of the tools at the Institute for Johns Hopkins Nursing Web site: www.ijhn.jhmi.edu

Johns Hopkins Nursing Evidence-Based Practice Model and Guidelines is a collaboration among three nurse leaders at The Johns Hopkins Hospital and two faculty members from The Johns Hopkins University School of Nursing. Developed and evaluated in multiple projects and settings, the JHNEBP Model and process is practical for organizations to implement. Additionally, it demystifies and enables the EBP process for bedside nurses. The JHNEBP Model won the Sigma Theta Tau International Research Utilization Award in 2005 at the 38th Biennial Convention in Indianapolis, Indiana.

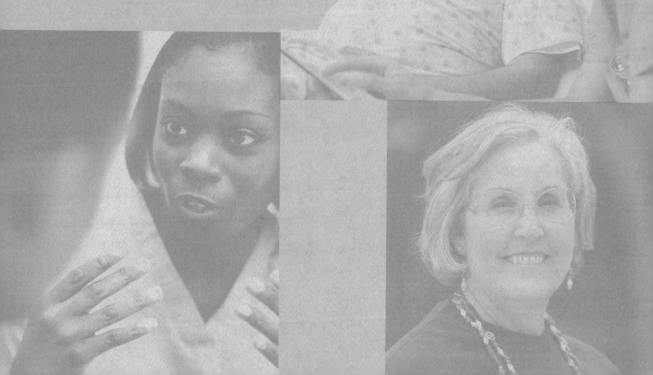

Evidence-Based Practice
Background

Chapter 1

Chapter 2

Evidence-Based Practice: Context, Concerns, and Challenges

Evidence-based practice (EBP) positions nurses to be a significant influence on health-care decisions and a partner in improving quality of care. Beyond an expectation for professional practice, EBP provides a major opportunity for nurses to enlighten practice and add value to the patient experience. Today, nursing interventions and processes informed by the best evidence are critical to realizing health-care improvements and cost savings. This chapter defines evidence-based practice and discusses the evolution of evidence-based practice within the nursing profession.

EBP: A Definition

EBP is a problem-solving approach to clinical decision making within a health-care organization that integrates the best available scientific evidence with the best available experiential (patient and practitioner) evidence. EBP considers internal and external influences on practice and encourages critical thinking in the judicious application of evidence to care of the individual patient, patient population, or system (Newhouse, Dearholt, Poe, Pugh, & White, 2005). EBP uses the latest research evidence to produce high-quality health care. The challenge for health-care providers is to implement the best interventions and practices informed by the evidence.

Key assumptions of evidence-based nursing practice include

1. Nursing is both a science and an applied profession.

2. Knowledge is important to professional practice, and there are limits to knowledge that must be identified.

3. Not all evidence is created equal, and there is a need to use the best available evidence.

4. Evidence-based practice contributes to improved outcomes (Newhouse, in press).

EBP supports and informs clinical, administrative, and educational decision making. Combining research, organizational experience (including quality improvement data and financial data), clinical expertise, expert opinion, and patient preferences ensures clinical decisions based on all available evidence. EBP ensures *efficacy* (the ability to reach a desired result), *efficiency* (the achievement of a desired result with a minimum of expense, time, and effort), and *effectiveness* (the ability to produce the desired result). Additionally, EBP weighs risk, benefit, and cost against a backdrop of patient preferences. This decision making encourages health-care providers to question practice and determine which interventions work and which do not. EBP ensures that nurses use evidence to promote optimal outcomes or equivalent care at lower cost or in less time and that health-care providers promote patient satisfaction and higher health-related quality of life.

EBP and Outcomes

Health-care providers by their nature have always been interested in the outcomes or results of a patient's care. Traditionally, the focus has been on morbidity and mortality. Today, the focus has broadened to include *clinical* (e.g., symptoms); *functional* (e.g., performance of daily activities); *quality of life* (e.g.

patient satisfaction); and *economic* (e.g., direct costs, indirect costs, intangible costs) outcomes. EBP conducts a critical review of how health-care practices and outcomes are linked, informing decisions that can result in quality of care improvements.

Governments and society challenge health-care providers to base their practices on current, validated interventions (Zerhouni, 2006). EBP can be seen as a response to this mandate, as well as a logical progression in the continuing effort to close the gap between research and practice (Stetler, 2001; Titler, Cullen, & Ardery, 2002; Weaver, Warren, & Delaney, 2005). Quality and cost concerns drive health care. Nurses, like other professionals, must operate within an *age of accountability* (McQueen & McCormick, 2001). This accountability has become a focal point for health care.

EBP and Accountability

Public expectations that health-care investments should consistently lead to high-quality results most likely will not diminish in the near future. Nowhere is accountability a more sensitive topic than in health care. Much of the information out there suggests consumers are not consistently receiving appropriate care (Institute of Medicine, 2001). It is within this environment that nurses, physicians, public health scientists, and others explore what works and what does not, and it is within this context that nurses and other health-care providers continue the journey to bridge research and practice.

EBP provides a systematic approach to decision making that achieves best practices and demonstrates accountability. When the strongest available evidence is considered, the odds of doing the right thing at the right time for the right patient are improved. Given the complexity of linking research and clinical practice, the definitions and concepts associated with EBP have developed over time and may vary according to the theoretical framework adopted. EBP provides a useful framework born of collaborative efforts to translate evidence into practice.

Translation involves the synthesis, implementation, evaluation, and dissemination of research and non-research evidence. EBP has evolved through the measurement of outcomes and the analysis of the overall conditions that foster individual patient and system-wide improvements. Nurses need to evaluate whether evidence from translation efforts provides needed insights that contribute to patient care, including whether best practice information (such as clinical practice guidelines) is useful when addressing complex clinical questions. Measuring these improvements and determining the best way to affect policy (if appropriate) are necessary. EBP depends on the collective capacity of nurses to develop cultures of critical thinking where ongoing learning is inherent. As the field evolves, nurses can serve patients and the profession by exploring translation processes and promoting the use of evidence in routine decisions.

The History

Although introducing new concepts and enhanced methods for research utilization, EBP is not conceptually new; its roots extend back many decades. However, the terms associated with any applied science change as the science evolves. In 1972, A. L. Cochrane, a British epidemiologist, criticized the health profession for not knowing the outcomes of medical treatment. In the 1980s, the term *evidence-based medicine* was being used at McMaster University Medical School in Canada. These events led to the establishment, in 1993, of the Cochrane Collaboration. The Cochrane Collaboration provides systematic reviews about the effects of health care. These reviews provide logical reasoning and sound evidence for providing effective treatment regimes.

Relatively new developments include: a) increasingly sophisticated analytical techniques; b) improved presentation and dissemination of information; c) growing knowledge of how to implement findings while effectively considering patient preferences, costs, and policy issues; and d) better understanding of how to measure effect and use feedback to promote ongoing improvement.

Knowing and Using Evidence

More is known than is practiced, and considerable delay exists in incorporating new knowledge into clinical practice. For example, in the 1970s, evidence supported the effectiveness of thrombolytic therapy in reducing mortality in acute myocardial infarction (Kiernan & Gersh, 2007), yet it is still not uniformly given in a timely way to patients who would benefit. New knowledge has grown exponentially. Early in the 20th century, there were few journals available, and they were not easily accessible to the professional nurse. Today, PubMed indexes 5,164 journals (National Library of Medicine, 2007). CINAHL (2006) indexes 1,839 journals. EBP is a strategy nurses can use to stay abreast of the explosion of new information.

There is also a decline in best care knowledge related to the amount of information available and the limited time to digest it. Studies show that knowledge of best care negatively correlates with year of graduation; that is, knowledge of best care practices declines as the number of years since graduation increases (Estabrooks, 1998; Shin, Haynes, & Johnson, 1993). Additionally, there is increasing consumer pressure to provide the most up-to-date therapies. The accessibility of information on the Web has increased consumer expectation of participating in treatment decisions. Patients with chronic health problems have accumulated considerable expertise in self-management, increasing the pressure for providers to be up-to-date with the best evidence for care.

Nursing Engages in Research Utilization

More than 30 years ago, the first major nurse-based EBP project began through the Western Interstate Commission for Higher Education (WICHE; Krueger, 1978). WICHE initiated the first attempt to use research in the clinical setting. A relatively new professional discipline, nursing was just beginning to develop and conduct research that was useful to clinicians. The outcomes of the 6-year WICHE project were not as favorable as anticipated. Nursing science targeted the study of nurses at the time, and finding interventions to use in practice was difficult.

The Conduct and Utilization of Research in Nursing Project (CURN) began in the 1970s (Horsley, Crane, & Bingle, 1978). There were 10 areas identified as having adequate evidence to use in practice (CURN Project, 1981-1982).

1. Structured preoperative teaching

2. Reducing diarrhea in tube-fed patients

3. Preoperative sensory preparation to promote recovery

4. Prevention of decubitus ulcers

5. Intravenous cannula change

6. Closed urinary drainage systems

7. Distress reduction through sensory preparation

8. Mutual goal setting in patient care

9. Clean intermittent catheterization

10. Pain: deliberate nursing interventions

In the 1980s, much attention focused on *research utilization* (RU). The National Institute of Nursing Research was developed, and attention to the research foundation of nursing became paramount. Teaching incorporated RU and some hospitals developed Centers for Nursing Research. Models to use research appeared, such as the Stetler Model (Stetler, 2001) and the Iowa Model (Titler et al., 2001). Increasingly, sophisticated nursing research and interventions based on rigorous research studies became the expectation.

The actual translation of research into practice has been slowly taking place since the 1960s. In 2000, Donaldson detailed the major scientific breakthroughs in health-care practice for the preceding 39-year period. See Table 1.1.

Table 1.1.   Examples of Translating Research Into Practice

Principal Scientist	Topic	Practice
Barbara Hanson	Gastrointestinal symptoms	Undesirable effects of lactose intolerance in patients receiving tube feedings are eliminated with the removal of lactose from these formulas.

Principal Scientist	Topic	Practice
Elizabeth Winslow	Cardiac precautions	Oxygen consumption and cardiovascular response during toileting were not different when toileting on a bedpan or using a bedside commode.
Jeanne Quint Benoliel	Personal experience of disease	Sharing the diagnosis and prognosis was not common in the early 1970s until these studies were widely disseminated.
Jean Johnson	Pain management	Distress symptoms lessen when children are prepared for the expected sensations that accompany cast removal.
Thelma Wells and Carol Brink	Stress urinary incontinence	Pelvic muscle exercises, as a self-care intervention, are effective in preventing stress urinary incontinence.

Examples adapted from Donaldson, S. K. (2000). Breakthroughs in scientific research: Discipline of nursing, 1960-1999. *Annual Review of Nursing Research, 18*, 247-311.

Differentiating RU and EBP

Since the introduction of EBP in the 1990s, questions regarding the relationship between RU and EBP have been raised. The terms are often used interchangeably; however, they are not synonymous. The two major differences: RU uses only research evidence (EBP incorporates non-research evidence), and RU is dependent on research publication and availability (EBP includes sources of data not yet published and organizational data). EBP incorporates theory, clinical decision making and judgment, and knowledge of research techniques, followed by application of the best, most effective, and clinically meaningful evidence (Melnyk & Fineout-Overholt, 2005). Evidence constitutes research findings as well as other sources of credible information, such as quality improvement data, operational data, evaluative data, consensus of experts, affirmed clinical experience, and patient preference. These other forms of evidence are combined with research findings to facilitate decision making or problem solving. RU uses the same critical review, recommendation, and implementation process as EBP.

Nursing's Role in EBP

EBP encompasses multiple sources of knowledge, clinical expertise, and patient preference. The evaluation, synthesis, and application of evidence may sometimes seem daunting. The nurse seeking the best available evidence at the bedside or policy table cannot expect to find easy answers. Nurses need to participate actively in how ideas surrounding the use of evidence evolve within the unit and organization. Nurses need to be active, skilled, and enlightened players. Managing the uncertainty that often surrounds clinical decisions is critical; nurses cannot afford to be intimidated or hesitant. Exploring ways to systematize the use of evidence (or deal with a lack of evidence) to promote optimal decisions excludes no source of knowledge or theory.

EBP integrates all decision makers who influence patient outcomes and system operation. Nurses are central to patient care and have strong incentives to use evidence and collaboration to support their decisions. Nurses have much to share and cannot afford to isolate themselves. Nursing as a profession has made a strong contribution to the collective understanding of how best to support decision making based on the best available evidence.

Summary

This chapter defines EBP and discusses the evolution that led to the critical need for practice based on evidence to guide decision making. EBP creates a culture of critical thinking and ongoing learning. It is the foundation for an environment where evidence supports clinical, administrative, and educational decisions. EBP supports rational decision making that reduces inappropriate variation and makes it easier for nurses to do their job.

Numbering more than 2 million and practicing in most health-care settings, nurses make up the largest number of health professionals. Every patient is likely to receive nursing care. Therefore, nurses are in an important position to influence the type, quality, and cost of care provided to patients.

For nursing, the framework for decision making has traditionally been the nursing process. Understood in this process is the use of assessment evidence to guide the nurse in planning care. EBP is an explicitly formal approach to enhancing efficiency. EBP facilitates meeting the needs of patients and delivering care that is effective, efficient, equitable, patient-centered, safe, and timely (Institute of Medicine, 2001).

References

Cochrane, A. L. (1972). *Effectiveness and efficiency: Random Reflections on health services.* London: Nuffield Provincial Hospitals Trust, Cochrane Collaboration.

Conduct and Utilization of Research in Nursing. (1981-1982). *Using research to improve nursing practice.* New York: Grune & Stratton.

Donaldson, S. K. (2000). Breakthroughs in scientific research: Discipline of nursing, 1960-1999. *Annual Review of Nursing Research, 18,* 247-311.

Estabrooks, C. A. (1998). Will evidence-based nursing practice make practice perfect? *Canadian Journal of Nursing Research, 30,* 15-36.

Horsley, J., Crane, J., & Bingle, J. (1978). Research utilization as an organizational process. *Journal of Nursing Administration, 8*(7), 4-6.

Institute of Medicine. (2001). *Crossing the Quality Chasm.* Washington, DC: National Academy Press.

Kiernan, T. J., & Gersh, B. J. (2007). Thrombolysis in acute myocardial infarction: Current status. *Medical Clinics of North America, 90,* 617-637.

Krueger, J. C. (1978). Utilization of nursing research: The planning process. *Journal of Nursing Administration, 8*(1), 6-9.

McQueen, L., & McCormick, K.A. (2001). Translating evidence into practice: Guidelines and automated implementation tools. In V. K. Saba & K. A. McCormick (Eds.), *Essentials of computers for nurses* (pp. 335-356), New York: McGraw Hill.

Melnyk, B. M., & Fineout-Overholt, E. (2005). *Evidence-based practice in nursing and health care: A guide to best practice.* Philadelphia: Lippincott, Williams & Wilkins.

National Library of Medicine. (2007). *List of journals indexed for MEDLINE.* Retrieved October 1, 2007, from http://www.nlm.nih.gov/tsd/serials/lji.html

Newhouse, R. P., Dearholt, S., Poe, S., Pugh, L. C., White, K. (2005). Evidence based practice: A practical approach to implementation. *Journal of Nursing Administration, 35*(1), 35-40.

Newhouse, R. P., Dearholt, S., Poe, S., Pugh, L. C., & White, K. (in press). Organizational change strategies for evidence-based practice. *Journal of Nursing Administration.*

Shin, J. H., Haynes, R. B., & Johnson, M. E. (1993). Effect of problem-based, self-directed education on life long learning. *Canadian Medical Association Journal, 148,* 969-976.

Stetler, C. (2001). *Evidence-based practice and the use of research: A synopsis of basic concepts & strategies to improve care.* Washington, DC: Nova Foundation.

Titler, M. G., Cullen, L., & Ardery, G. (2002). Evidence-based practice: An administrative perspective. *Reflections on Nursing Leadership, 28,* 26-27.

Titler, M. G., Kleiber, C, Steelman, V. J., Rakel, B. A., Budreau, G, Everett L. Q., et al. (2001). The Iowa Model of evidence-based practice to promote quality care. *Critical Care Nursing Clinics North America, 13,* 497-509.

Weaver, C., Warren, J. J., & Delaney, C. (2005). Bedside, classroom and bench: Collaborative strategies to generate evidence-based knowledge for nursing practice. *International Journal of Medical Informatics, 74,* 989-999.

Zerhouni, E. (2006). Research funding. NIH in the post doubling era: Realities and strategies. *Science, 314,* 1088-1090.

Other Resources

Wennberg, D. E., & Wennberg, J.E. (2003). Addressing variations: Is there hope for the future? *Health Affairs*, W3-614-7. Retrieved October 1, 2007, from http://content.healthaffairs.org/cgi/reprint/hlthaff.w3.614v1

Wennberg, J. E. (1996). Practice variations and the challenge to leadership. *Spine*, *21*, 1472-1478.

Wennberg, J. E., & Fowler, F. J. (1977). A test of consumer contribution to small area variations in health care delivery. *Journal of the Maine Medical Assocoiation*, 68(8), 275-279.

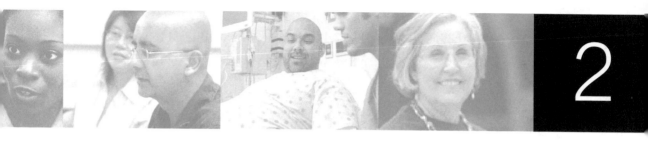

Critical Thinking and Evidence-Based Practice

The very nature of nursing practice compels nurses to play an active role in advancing best practices in patient care. Professional practice involves making judgments; without judgment, professional practice is merely technical work (Coles, 2002). Professional judgment is enabled by critical thinking. There are many definitions of critical thinking found in the literature; however, the complexity of this process requires explanation rather than definition (Riddell, 2007).

Critical thinking is a complex cognitive process that involves questioning, seeking information, analyzing, synthesizing, drawing conclusions from available information, and transforming knowledge into action (American Association of Colleges of Nursing, 1998; Scheffer & Rubenfeld, 2000). Critical thinking is a dynamic process that serves as the foundation of clinical reasoning and decision making and, as such, is a critical component of developing evidence-based practice. Each clinical scenario provides the nurse with an opportunity to use acquired knowledge and skills to provide care that is effective for the particular individual, family, or group (Dickerson, 2005). Regardless of the nature or the source of evidence used by nurses to support patient care, critical thinking supplies the necessary skills and cognitive habits required to support evidence-based practice (Profetto-McGrath, 2005).

Practicing nurses, as well as their nurse leaders, may find that the demands of myriad patient-care tasks can create a shift in focus away from use of critical thinking skills. This chapter provides nurse leaders with the knowledge and skills needed to foster critical thinking to support the activities of evidence-based practice. The chapter's specific objectives are to:

- illustrate the similarities between evidence-based practice and the nursing process

- establish critical thinking skills as essential to the nursing process and evidence-based practice

- discuss the role of critical thinking in the Practice question, Evidence, and Translation process

This chapter closes with recommendations to clinical nurse leaders to help champion critical thinking skills as a key component of evidence-based practice.

Evidence and the Nursing Process

Evidence-based practice (EBP) has an evolving nature; consequently, what constitutes evidence continues to advance over time. Nurses, as key members of interdisciplinary teams, already have the will and the determination to participate in a meaningful way in the advancement of best practices in patient care. What they may not possess, however, are the skills to pose an answerable practice question, gather and critically appraise evidence that may provide the response to that question, or logically reason whether to translate relevant findings into practice. These skills are prerequisites to informed decision making about the application of best practices to the care of individual patients.

The American Nurses Association (ANA) Standards of Nursing Practice (2004) lists each step of the nursing process, from collection of comprehensive data pertinent to the patient's health or situation through evaluation of the outcomes of planned interventions. The ANA Standards of Professional Performance (2004) contains the integration of the best available evidence, including research findings, to guide practice decisions. These standards contribute to the overall problem-solving strategy that frames patient-care decision making.

The similarity between EBP and the nursing process has been noted (Sharts-Hopko, 2003). Both are problem-solving strategies. The nursing process structures nursing practice through the following problem-solving stages: *assessment, diagnosis, outcome identification, planning, intervention,* and *evaluation.* Although critical thinking is thought to be inherent in the nursing process, this has not been empirically demonstrated (Fesler-Birch, 2005). Nevertheless, the nursing process does require certain skills that are also necessary for critical thinking, such as seeking information and synthesizing (assessment), drawing conclusions from available information (diagnosis), and transforming knowledge into an action plan (planning). The concept of critical thinking, however, extends beyond the well-defined nursing process (Tanner, 2000).

The Practice question, Evidence, and Translation process (PET) structures the activities of EBP. The nurse asks a focused clinical question, searches for relevant evidence, analyzes the evidence, uses the evidence in patient care, and evaluates the outcome (Stuart, 2001). After identifying the practice question (P), the nurse enters into the evidence (E) phase, and then finally, the translation (T) phase. Each phase requires an analogous set of critical thinking skills including questioning, information seeking, synthesizing, logical reasoning, and transforming knowledge.

Carper (1978) defined four patterns of knowing in nursing: *empirical* (the science of nursing), *ethical* (the code of nursing), *personal* (knowledge gained from interpersonal relationships between nurse and patient), and *aesthetic* (the art of nursing). Each of these aspects contributes to the body of evidence on which practice is based. Building on Carper's work, McKenna, Cutcliffe, and McKenna (2000) postulated that there are four types of evidence to consider:

- *empirical evidence:* evidence based on scientific research

- *ethical evidence:* evidence based on the nurse's knowledge of and respect for the patient's values and preferences

■ *personal evidence:* evidence based on the nurse's experience in caring for the particular patient

■ *aesthetic evidence:* evidence based on the nurse's intuition, interpretation, understanding, and personal values

It is the compilation and critical appraisal of all types of evidence, alone and as they relate to each other, that results in the nurse's decision to adopt or reject evidence in the care of the particular patient.

The Johns Hopkins Nursing Evidence-based Practice Model (JHNEBP) broadly categorizes evidence as either research or non-research. Scientific, or empirical, evidence remains a separate category, research, whereas non-research evidence comprises ethical, personal, and aesthetic evidence. Inherent in the JHNEBP Model's definition of EBP is the relationship between critical thinking and the judicious application of evidence to care through the PET process.

Critical Thinking and EBP

Confucius (500 BC) wrote: "Shall I teach you what knowledge is? When you know a thing, to hold that you know it; and when you do not know a thing, to allow that you do not know it—this is knowledge." This maxim can be applied to contemporary nursing practice and lays the foundation for the role of critical thinking in EBP. Whittemore (1999) interprets this teaching as, "to know is to act knowledge" and adds: "Acting knowledge is the outcome of the integration of multiple perceptions, thoughts, and critical analysis in any given experience. It is the translation of what one knows into what one does" (p. 365). That is, the integration of scientific and non-research knowledge that occurs during the critical appraisal process actually enables such translation into everyday nursing practice.

Many of today's novice nurses appear to concentrate primarily on tasks, focusing on the "how" of nursing care. This is an expected consequence as new nurses transition into the work environment with myriad newly acquired technical skills. The focus on tasks does not encourage reflection on the who, what, where, when, and why of care. Even more experienced nurses find themselves refraining from asking "why" as they become embroiled in responsibilities beyond their individual patient-care assignments. EBP not only directs nurses to ask "why," but also helps them to frame the answer to the question so that patient-care decisions are made with reflection and deliberation.

The concept of *reflection* in clinical practice as it relates to developing expertise is not unique to nursing. Reflection, a key cognitive mechanism in critical thinking, allows the nurse to create and clarify the meaning of a particular experience (Forneris & Peden-McAlpine, 2007). Reflection in the context of nursing practice "is viewed as a process of transforming unconscious types of knowledge and practices into conscious, explicit, and logically articulated knowledge and practices that allows for transparent and justifiable clinical decision making" (Mantzoukas, 2007, p. 7).

In her landmark book, originally published in 1985, Benner (2001) applied the Dreyfus Model of Skill Acquisition (Dreyfus & Dreyfus, 1986) to the professional development of nurses. Progressing through the stages of novice to expert, nurses learn to link the technical aspect of expertise with the intuitive aspect of expertise. That is, to manage patient-care situations, nurses refine their critical thinking skills to integrate experience with acquired knowledge.

Paul and Elder (1996a) suggest that to think critically requires having command of the following universal intellectual standards: Clarity, Accuracy, Precision, Relevance, Depth, Breadth, and Logic. These intellectual standards can be invaluable to members of the EBP team. If a statement is unclear, the team cannot judge the accuracy or relevance of the statement to the practice question. Similarly, superficial answers or those that present only one point of view do not address the complexities of most health-care questions. Finally, after developing a well-reasoned answer, team members need to decide whether the answer is practical for translation into practice for the particular patient population.

The Assessment Technologies Institute (ATI), a nurse educator-run testing company that serves schools of nursing throughout the country, developed the Critical Thinking Assessment (CTA)—a scientifically normalized and validated critical thinking appraisal tool (Whitehead, 2006). The 40-item CTA addresses six competencies to measure critical thinking (Assessment Technologies Institute, 2006):

- *interpretation*: the ability to comprehend and identify problems

- *analysis*: the ability to inspect, organize, categorize, discriminate among, and prioritize variables

- *evaluation*: the ability to assess integrity, significance, and applicability of sources of information needed to support conclusions

- *inference*: the ability to develop hypotheses or draw conclusions based on evidence

- *explanation*: the ability to clarify assumptions that lead to conclusions reached

- *self-regulation*: the ability to examine and correct one's actions

Other educators have postulated cognitive critical thinking skills that validate and augment those in the CTA. Taylor-Seehafer, Abel, Tyler, and Sonstein (2004) proposed the importance of the following core cognitive skills in the education of nurse practitioners:

- *divergent thinking*: the ability to analyze a variety of opinions

- *reasoning*: the ability to differentiate between fact and conjecture

- *reflection*: time to deliberate and identify multidimensional processes

- *creativity*: considering multiple solutions

- *clarification*: noting similarities, differences, and assumptions

- *basic support*: evaluating credibility of sources of information

Much has been written regarding proposed characteristics of critical thinkers. Beyond the requisite knowledge and skills, critical thinkers must have the necessary attitudes, attributes, and habits of mind to use this knowledge and complement these skills (Profetto-McGrath, 2005). One approach to defining these basic dispositions proposes that there are certain *intellectual virtues* that are valuable to the critical thinker (Foundation for Critical Thinking, 1996). A second approach identifies *habits of the mind* exhibited by critical thinkers (Scheffer & Rubenfeld, 2000). Table 2.1 outlines these two complementary disposition sets. When participating in

EBP projects, the team should be aware of these intellectual virtues and habits of the mind to avoid the pitfalls of vague, fragmented, or close-minded thinking.

Table 2.1. Attributes of Critical Thinkers

Intellectual Virtues of Critical Thinkers[1]	Habits of Mind of Critical Thinkers[2]
■ Intellectual Humility: being aware of the limits of one's knowledge	■ Confidence: assurance of one's own ability to reason
■ Intellectual Courage: being open and fair when addressing ideas, viewpoints, or beliefs that differ from one's own	■ Contextual Perspective: ability to consider the whole in its entirety
■ Intellectual Empathy: being aware of the need to put one's self in another's place to achieve genuine understanding	■ Creativity: intellectual inventiveness ■ Flexibility: capacity to adapt
■ Intellectual Integrity: holding one's self to the same rigorous standards of evidence and proof as one does others	■ Inquisitiveness: seeking knowledge and understanding through thoughtful questioning and observation
■ Intellectual Perseverance: being cognizant of the need to use rational principles despite obstacles to doing so	■ Intellectual Integrity: seeking truth, even if results are contrary to one's assumptions or beliefs
■ Faith in Reason: being confident that people can learn to critically think for themselves	■ Intuition: sense of knowing without conscious use of reason
■ Fair-mindedness: understanding that one needs to treat all viewpoints in an unbiased fashion	■ Open-mindedness: receptivity to divergent views
	■ Perseverance: determination to stay on course
	■ Reflection: contemplation for deeper understanding and self-evaluation

[1] The Foundation for Critical Thinking, 1996
[2] Scheffer and Rubenfeld, 2000

Cultivating critical thinking skills in nursing students and practicing nurses at all levels has been a key concern for nursing educators and nurse administrators (Chen & Lin, 2003; Eisenhauer, Hurley, & Dolan, 2007). Due to the unpredictable nature of clinical nursing care, nurses need the ability to analyze and interpret cues, weigh evidence, and respond appropriately and promptly to changing clinical situations requiring immediate action (Greenwood, Sullivan, Spence, & McDonald, 2000). This ability to think critically is a valuable asset to the nurse member of the EBP team when evaluating the cumulative body of evidence for its potential applicability to particular patient-care situations.

Critical Thinking and the PET Process

Critical Thinking and the Practice Question

The first step to translating evidence into practice requires the ability to pose an answerable *practice question*. Questioning is key to critical thinking. Questions determine what information to seek and the direction in which to search. Asking a well-built question may be more challenging than answering the question itself (Schlosser, Koul, & Costello, 2007).

Universal intellectual standards (clarity, accuracy, precision, relevance, breadth, and logic) can assist in determining the quality of reasoning about a problem, issue, or situation (Paul & Elder, 1996b). These standards can be applied to the practice question to refine that question. The practice question should be clear, accurate, precise, and relevant. If the question posed is unclear or is based on a false assumption, it may not be truly reflective of the issue under investigation. If the practice question is unspecific, it may not contain sufficient detail to be answerable. If the practice question is irrelevant to the concern, the EBP team will find it difficult to gather evidence that provides an appropriate answer. The question should have enough depth and breadth to consider the complexities of care, but should not be so broad that the search for evidence becomes too difficult to manage. Finally, the question needs to make sense and contain no contradictory elements.

The use of critical thinking skills is not limited to development of the practice question; critical thinking skills are also important to conducting the remaining steps of the practice question phase. Defining the scope of the problem entails that the nurse consider the whole situation, including background and environment relevant to the phenomenon of interest. Project leaders and interdisciplinary team members need to possess intellectual habits attributable to critical thinkers. These habits include confidence, creativity, flexibility, inquisitiveness, intellectual integrity, and open-mindedness. Having members who are flexible and determined enhances a team's ability to meet the most difficult challenges, as scheduling meetings can be difficult in the best of circumstances.

The nursing practice environment provides the source of most EBP questions. Issues prompting inquiry can arise from a multitude of sources, including safety/risk management concerns, unsatisfactory patient outcomes, wide variations in practice, significant financial or cost concerns, differences between hospital and community practice, clinical practice issues of concern, procedures or processes that waste time, or practices with no scientific basis.

Schlosser, Koul, and Costello (2007, p. 227) proposed, "The process of asking well-built questions should be formalized, such that the ingredients of a well-built question are known, and well-built questions can be distinguished from poorly stated questions." The JHNEBP Model uses a question development tool (see Appendix A) to serve as a guide for generating useful questions and defining the scope of the problem. Components of this tool as they relate to critical thinking standards are outlined in Table 2.2. The PICO organizing template (Richardson, Wilson, Nishikawa, & Hayward, 1995) is used to structure question development and is discussed in more detail in Chapter 4.

Table 2.2.   Practice Question Development and Critical Thinking Standards

Practice Question Components	Critical Thinking Standards and Questions
What is the practice issue?	*Clarity:* Is the issue clear? Can we give an example?
What is the current practice?	
How was the practice issue identified?	*Accuracy:* Is it true because we believe it, we want to believe it, we have always believed it, or it is in our vested interest to believe it?
What are the PICO components? (patient/population/problem, intervention, comparison with other treatments if applicable, outcome)	*Precision:* Can we provide more detail on the issue? What is the issue? What intervention are we questioning? Do we wish to compare this with some other intervention?
	Logic: What is our desired outcome? Does it really make sense?

Table 2.2.   Practice Question Development and Critical Thinking Standards (continued)

Practice Question Components	Critical Thinking Standards and Questions
State the search question in narrow, manageable terms.	*Precision*: Can we be more specific?
What evidence must be gathered?	*Relevance*: How is this evidence connected to the question? Are we addressing the most significant factors related to the question?
State the search strategy, database, and key words.	*Breadth*: Do we need to consider other points of view? Are there other ways to look at the question?

Critical Thinking and Evidence

The *evidence* phase of the PET process requires proficiency in the following critical thinking skills: *seeking information, analyzing, synthesizing, interpreting,* and *drawing conclusions from available information.* The critical analysis, synthesis, and interpretation of evidence are made explicit by the use of rating scales. These scales provide a structured way to enhance the critical thinking skills of the nurse reviewer by facilitating the assignment of standardized levels to evidence, to differentiate among evidence of varying strengths and quality. The underlying assumption is that recommendations from strong evidence of high quality would be more likely to represent best practices than evidence of lower strength and less quality. Appendix B depicts the rating scale used in the JHNEBP Model to determine strength of evidence.

Scientific evidence is generally given a higher strength rating than is non-research evidence, in particular when the scientific evidence is of high quality. To apply critical thinking skills when appraising scientific research, the nurse looks at two major components when evaluating individual studies: *study design* (usually classified as experimental, quasi-experimental, non-experimental and qualitative) and *study quality* (evaluation of study methods and procedure). When evaluating the summary of overall evidence, there are four major components: *study design, quality, consistency* (similarities in the size and/or direction of estimated effects across studies), and *directness* (the extent to which subjects, interventions, and outcome measures are similar to those of interest) (GRADE Working Group, 2004). Chapter 6 presents the various types of research evidence and their associated levels of evidential strength.

Because of the complex human and environmental context of nursing care, research evidence is not sufficient to inform practice. In many instances, scientific evidence either does not exist or is insufficient to inform nursing practice for the individual patient, population, or system. Non-research evidence is then needed to inform nursing knowledge. Evidence derived from sources other than research generally includes summaries of research evidence reports, expert opinion, practitioner experience and expertise, patient experience, and human/organizational experience. Critical appraisal of the strength of non-research evidence is not as well established as scientific evidence and is, therefore, more challenging. Because non-research evidence is thought to be outside the realm of science, appraisal methods have rarely been considered. Chapter 7 discusses the various types of non-research evidence and their use either in lieu of or as an adjunct to research evidence.

The large number of checklists, scales, and similar tools available for grading the quality of individual reports complicates how the nurse reviewer applies critical thinking skills to grade the quality of publications used for evidence-based decision making (Lohr & Carey, 1999). Most of these tools are designed to assess the quality of research evidence. Similar to the appraisal of evidence strength, the appraisal of the quality of non-research evidence is not well defined. Tools to appraise research evidence usually contain explicit criteria for review of quality, with varying degrees of specificity to the type of scientific evidence under review. Nurses without graduate degrees generally do not have the comprehensive methodological knowledge of strengths and limitations required to interpret these criteria.

The development of any EBP skill set is an evolutionary process. Critical thinking is thought to be "a lifelong process requiring self-awareness, knowledge, and practice" (Brunt, 2005, p. 66). The JHNEBP Model uses a broadly defined quality rating scale to provide some degree of structure for the nurse reviewer, yet allows for the application of critical thinking skills specific to the knowledge and experience of the team reviewing the evidence. This scale is represented in Appendix B. The application of this scale accommodates qualitative judgments related to both scientific and non-research evidence.

Judgments of quality should be continually approached in relative terms. The EBP team assigns a quality grade for each piece of evidence reviewed. The judgment that underlies this determination is in relation to the body of past and present evidence that each member has reviewed. As the group and its individual members gain experience reading and appraising research, their abilities and judgments will likely improve.

Critical Thinking and Translation

The challenge for a nurse participating in EBP is combining the contributions of each type of evidence (research and non-research) when making patient-care decisions. Not only must the nurse grade the strength and quality of evidence, but he or she must also determine the compatibility of recommendations with the patient's values and preferences and the clinician's expertise (Melnyk & Fineout-Overholt, 2006).

Two goals of critical thinking are to assess credibility of information and to work through problems to make decisions in the best way (Halpern, 1996). This requires flexibility, persistence, and self-awareness on the part of the nurse. It challenges the nurse to consider alternate ways of thinking and acting. Maudsley and Strivens (2000), writing on critical thinking for tomorrow's doctors, postulated that a competent practitioner must use critical thinking skills to appraise evidence, tempering realistic notions of scientific evidence with a healthy dose of reflective skepticism. This also holds true for nurses as they execute the translation phase of evidence-based practice.

Recommendations for Nurse Leaders

While there are key elements of critical thinking not discussed within the context of the nursing process, there is no doubt that components of critical thinking are vital to the work of nursing. Therefore, nursing accreditation bodies recognize critical thinking as "a significant outcome for graduates at the baccalaureate and master's levels" (Ali, Bantz, & Siktberg, 2005, p. 90). Furthermore, critical thinking skills, such as questioning, analyzing, synthesizing, and drawing conclusions from available information, are definite assets to the nurse's ability to conduct meaningful evidence-based practice decisions.

Senge (1990) described *team learning*—the interaction of a team to produce learning and solve problems—as an essential component of his *learning organizations* concept, in which leaders continuously develop capacity for the future. Building capacity for nurses to carry out EBP projects is of strategic importance for nurse leaders. Therefore, ensuring that these nurses have the knowledge and skills required to procure and judge the value of evidence is a top leadership priority.

One way to achieve the successful cultural transition to evidence-based practice is to apply the notion of interactive team learning (Sams, Penn, & Facteau, 2004). As members of the EBP team gain experience reviewing and critiquing both research and non-research evidence related to a clinical question of interest to them, their motivation to integrate evidence into practice will increase. In order to do so, it is essential that nurses have a sound knowledge base regarding the nature of research and non-research evidence.

Nurse leaders can best support EBP by providing clinicians with the knowledge and skills necessary to pose answerable questions, to seek and appraise scientific and other quantitative and qualitative evidence within the context of non-research evidence, and to make a determination on the advisability of translating evidence into practice. Only through continuous learning can clinicians gain the confidence needed to incorporate the broad range of evidence into development of protocols and care standards as well as the personalized care of individual patients. Additionally, nurse educators can advance EBP by including related skill development as part of the nursing curricula. This will provide a larger pool from which nurse leaders can draw potential employees with a strong educational background in EBP.

Summary

This chapter describes the knowledge and skills needed to foster critical thinking to support EBP activities. Similarities between EBP and the nursing process, and the essential nature of the relationships between critical thinking, EBP, and the nursing process are discussed. Specific examples of the role of critical thinking in each phase of the Practice question, Evidence, and Translation process (PET) are provided.

In today's dynamic health-care environment, nurses cannot achieve expertise without maintaining continual awareness of the entire realm of known research (Pape, 2003). It is virtually impossible for staff nurses to give their complete attention to keeping track of all studies relevant to their practice. Knowledge gained through expensive, professional education coupled with non-research learning guide much of the nurse's practice.

Valid clinical questions arise during the course of the nurse's day-to-day patient-care activities. These are the questions that form the basis for many EBP projects, which benefit from the combined critical thinking of collaborative teams of nurses and their interdisciplinary colleagues. As Scheffer and Rubenfeld (2006, page 195) eloquently stated, "Putting the critical thinking dimensions into the development of evidence-based practice competency demonstrates how critical thinking can be taken out of the toolbox and used in the real world."

References

Ali, N. S., Bantz, D., & Siktberg, L. (2005). Validation of critical thinking skills in online responses. *Journal of Nursing Education, 44*(2), 90-94.

American Association of Colleges of Nursing. (1998). *The essentials of baccalaureate education for professional nursing practice.* Washington, DC: Author.

American Nurses Association. (2004). *Nursing: Scope and standards of practice.* Washington, DC: Author.

Assessment Technologies Institute. (2003). *The critical thinking assessment technical report.* Assessment Technologies Institute, LLC, Overland Park, Kansas. Retrieved October 19, 2007, from http://www.atitesting.com

Benner, P. E. (2001). *From novice to expert: Excellence and power in clinical nursing practice. Commemorative edition.* Upper Saddle River, NJ: Prentice Hall.

Brunt, B. A. (2005). Critical thinking in nursing: An integrated review. *The Journal of Continuing Education in Nursing, 36*, 60-67.

Carper, B. (1978). Fundamental patterns of knowing in nursing. *ANS. Advances in Nursing Science, 1*(1), 13-23.

Chen, F. C., & Lin, M. C. (2003). Effects of a nursing literature reading course on promoting critical thinking in two-year nursing program students. *Journal of Nursing Research, 11*(2), 137-146.

Coles, C. (2002). Developing professional judgment. *Journal of Continuing Education, 22*(1), 3-11.

Confucius. (500 B.C.). *The Analects* (Book 2, Chapter 17). English translation by James Legge. Retrieved February 28, 2005, from http://nothingistic.org/library/confucius/analects/

Dickerson, P. S. (2005). Nurturing critical thinkers. *The Journal of Continuing Education in Nursing, 36*(2), 68-72.

Dreyfus, H. L., & Dreyfus, S. E. (1986). *Mind over machine.* New York, NY: The Free Press.

Eisenhauer, L. A., Hurley, A.C., & Dolan, N. (2007). Nurses' reported thinking during medication administration. *Journal of Nursing Scholarship, 39,* 82-87.

Fesler-Birch, D. M. (2005). Critical thinking and patient outcomes: A review. *Nursing Outlook, 53,* 59-65.

Forneris, S. G., & Peden-McAlpine, C. (2007). Evaluation of a reflective learning intervention to improve critical thinking in novice nurses. *Journal of Advanced Nursing, 57,* 410-421.

Foundation for Critical Thinking. (1996). *Valuable intellectual virtues.* Retrieved August 30, 2006, from http://criticalthinking.org/resources/articles/

GRADE Working Group. (2004). Grading quality of evidence and strength of recommendations. *British Medical Journal, 328,* 1490-1498.

Greenwood, J., Sullivan, J., Spence, K., & McDonald, M. (2000). Nursing scripts and the organizational influences on critical thinking: Report of a study of neonatal nurses' clinical reasoning. *Journal of Advanced Nursing, 31,* 1106-1114.

Halpern, D. F. (1996). *Thought and knowledge: An introduction to critical thinking* (3rd ed.). Mahwah, NJ: Erlbaum.

Lohr, K. N., & Carey, T. S. (1999). Assessing "best evidence": Issues in grading the quality of studies for systematic reviews. *The Joint Commission Journal on Quality Improvement, 25*(9), 470-479.

Mantzoukas, S. (2007). A review of evidence-based practice, nursing research, and reflection: Leveling the hierarchy. *Journal of Clinical Nursing* (OnlineEarly Articles). Retrieved October 19, 2007, from http://www.blackwell-synergy.com/toc/jcn/0/0

Maudsley, G., & Strivens, J. (2000). 'Science,' 'critical thinking,' and 'competence' for tomorrow's doctors. A review of terms and concepts. *Medical Education, 34,* 53-60.

McKenna, H., Cutcliffe, J., & McKenna, P. (2000). Evidence-based practice: Demolishing some myths. *Nursing Standard, 14*(16), 39-42.

Melnyk, B. M., & Fineout-Overholt, E. (2006). Consumer preferences and values as an integral key to evidence-based practice. *Nursing Administration Quarterly, 30*(2), 123-127.

Pape, T. M. (2003). Evidence-based nursing practice: To infinity and beyond. *The Journal of Continuing Education in Nursing, 34*(4), 154-161.

Paul, R., & Elder, L. (1996a). *Universal intellectual standards*. Retrieved August 30, 2006, from http://criticalthinking.org/resources/articles/

Paul, R., & Elder, L. (1996b). *The critical mind is a questioning mind*. Retrieved August 30, 2006, from http://criticalthinking.org/resources/articles/

Profetto-McGrath, J. (2005). Critical thinking and evidence-based practice. *Journal of Professional Nursing, 21*(6), 364-371.

Richardson, W., Wilson, M., Nishikawa, J., & Hayward, R. (1995). The well-built clinical question: a key to evidence-based decisions. *ACP Journal Club, 123,* A12-A13.

Riddell, T. (2007). Critical assumptions: Thinking critically about critical thinking. *Journal of Nursing Education, 46*(3), 121-126.

Sams, L., Penn, B. K., & Facteau, L. (2004). The challenge of using evidence-based practice. *Journal of Nursing Administration, 34*(9), 407-414.

Scheffer, B., & Rubenfeld, G. (2000). A consensus statement on critical thinking in nursing. *Journal of Nursing Education, 39*(8), 352-359.

Scheffer, B. K., & Rubenfeld, M. G. (2006). Critical thinking: A tool in search of a job. *Journal of Nursing Education, 45,* 195-196.

Schlosser, R. W., Koul, R., & Costello, J. (2007). Asking well-built questions for evidence-based practice in augmentative and alternative communication. *Journal of Communication Disorders, 40*(3), 225-238.

Senge, P. M. (1990). *The fifth discipline. The art and practice of the learning organization.* New York: Doubleday.

Sharts-Hopko, N. C. (2003). Evidence-based practice: What constitutes evidence? *Journal of the Association of Nurses in Aids Care, 14*(3), 76-78.

Stuart, G. W. (2001). Evidence-based psychiatric nursing practice: Rhetoric or reality. *Journal of the American Psychiatric Nurses Association, 7,* 103-111.

Tanner, C. A. (2000). Critical thinking: Beyond nursing process. *Journal of Nursing Education, 39,* 338-339.

Taylor-Seehafer, M. A., Abel, E., Tyler, D. O., & Sonstein, F. C. (2004). Integrating evidence-based practice in nurse practitioner education. *Journal of the American Academy of Nurse Practitioners, 16*(12), 520-525.

Whitehead, T. D. (2006). Comparison of native versus nonnative English-speaking nurses on critical thinking assessments at entry and exit. *Nursing Administration Quarterly, 30,* 285-290.

Whittemore, R. (1999). To know is to act knowledge: Analects 2, 17. *Image: Journal of Nursing Scholarship, 31*(4), 365-366.

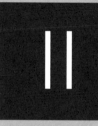

The Johns Hopkins
Evidence-Based Practice
Model and Guidelines

Chapter 3

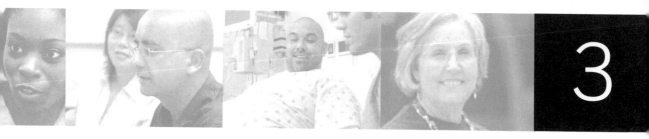

The Johns Hopkins Nursing Evidence-Based Practice Model and Process Overview

Nursing is a truly multidimensional profession. "Nursing is the protection, promotion, and optimization of health and abilities, prevention of illness and injury, alleviation of suffering through the diagnosis and treatment of human response, and advocacy in the care of individuals, families, communities and populations" (American Nurses Association, 2004, p. 7). Nurses work individually and as members of the health-care team, working collaboratively and in consultation with other health-care professionals, such as physicians, pharmacists, social workers, respiratory therapists, and physical therapists. Nurses strive to provide the highest quality nursing care that yields the best patient outcomes in today's financially constrained health-care environment. Critical thinking skills (see Chapter 2) applied to the evaluation of scientific and best available evidence, and subsequent application to nursing practice, assist in meeting this goal by helping to optimize patient outcomes based on best practices. This chapter describes the Johns Hopkins Nursing Evidence-Based Practice Model and introduces the Practice question, Evidence, and Translation process.

The Johns Hopkins Nursing Evidence-Based Practice Model

The Johns Hopkins Nursing Evidence-Based Practice Model (JHNEBP) (see Appendix C) depicts three essential cornerstones that form the foundation for professional nursing. These cornerstones are practice, education, and research. *Practice* is the basic component of all nursing activity (Porter-O'Grady, 1984). Nursing practice is the means by which a patient receives nursing care. It is an integral component of health-care organizations. *Education* reflects the acquisition of the nursing knowledge and skills necessary to become a proficient clinician and to maintain competency. *Research* provides new knowledge to the profession and enables the development of practices based on scientific evidence.

Nursing Practice

Nursing standards of care (protocols and procedures), *standards of practice* (professional standards), and the *nursing process* comprise the major components of nursing practice. The American Nurses Association (2004) has identified six standards of nursing practice incorporating the nursing process (see Table 3.1) and nine standards of professional performance (see Table 3.2).

Table 3.1.   American Nurses Association Standards of Practice (2004)

1. *Assessment:* the collection of comprehensive data pertinent to the patient's health or the situation. Data collection should be systematic and ongoing. As applicable, evidence-based assessment tools or instruments should be used—for example, evidence-based fall assessment tool, pain rating scales, or wound assessment tools.

2. *Diagnosis:* the analysis of assessment data to determine the diagnoses or issues.

3. *Outcomes identification:* the identification of expected outcomes for a plan individualized to the patient or the situation. Associated risks, benefits, costs, current scientific evidence, and clinical expertise should be considered when formulating expected outcomes.

4. *Planning:* the development of a plan that prescribes strategies and alternatives to attain expected outcomes. The plan should reflect current research and other evidence that are relevant to the planning process.

5. *Implementation:* execution of the identified plan, which includes the coordination and documentation of the plan and the care provided, teaching to promote health, and patient safety and consultation to influence the identified plan, enhance the abilities of others and to effect change.

6. *Evaluation:* progress toward attainment of outcomes. The evaluation should be systematic, ongoing, and criterion-based, and should include an indicated time-line.

Table 3.2. American Nurses Association Professional Performance Standards (2004)

1. *Quality of practice:* systematically enhancing the quality and effectiveness of nursing practice. Includes use of quality improvement and existing evidence to improve or initiate changes in nursing practice.

2. *Education:* attaining knowledge and competency that reflect current nursing practice. Commitment to lifelong learning and identifying learning needs.

3. *Professional practice evaluation:* evaluation of one's nursing practice in relation to professional practice standards and guidelines, relevant statutes, rules, and regulations.

4. *Collegiality:* interacting and contributing to the professional development of peers and colleagues.

5. *Collaboration:* partnering with the patient, family, and others (such as the multidisciplinary team) in the conduct of nursing practice to effect change and improve patient outcomes.

6. *Ethics:* the integration of ethical provisions in all areas of practice and the delivery of care in a manner that preserves and protects patient autonomy, dignity, and rights.

7. *Research:* the integration of research findings into practice by utilizing the best available evidence to guide practice decisions.

8. *Resource Utilization:* considers factors related to safety, effectiveness, cost, and impact on practice in the planning and delivering of nursing services.

9. *Leadership:* providing leadership in the professional practice setting and the profession.

Traditionally, much of nursing practice has been based on expert opinion and historic practice. Even today, nursing interventions can be identified that have little or no research to support the practices or to support their use over other interventions. An organizational approach designed to promote the questioning of nursing practice by nurses, and the use of EBP to answer these questions, serves to validate current practice or indicate the need to change practice based on evidence.

Additionally, an organization's ability to create opportunities for nurses to work within an interdisciplinary team to develop EBP questions, evaluate evidence, and make practice changes helps to build critical thinking skills and promotes professional development. In our experience, nursing staff members who participate in the EBP process report feeling greater autonomy and satisfaction as a result of contributing to changes in nursing practice based on evidence. Change may also be more readily accepted in the organization and by other disciplines when it is based on evidence that has been evaluated through the EBP process.

Nursing Education

Nursing education begins with basic education (generally an associate or baccalaureate degree) in which fundamental nursing skills and knowledge, natural and behavioral sciences, professional values, behaviors, and attitudes are learned. Advanced education (master's or doctorate degree) expands knowledge, refines practice, and often leads to specialization in a particular practice area. Advanced nursing education incorporates an increased emphasis on the application of research and other types of evidence to influence or change nursing practice.

In addition to formal education, ongoing education, such as conferences, seminars, workshops, and inservices, is required in order to keep current with new knowledge, technologies, and skills, or to establish initial and ongoing clinical competencies. Education is also gained from nursing practice and experience, leading to the development of critical thinking skills and enhancing the individual nurse's ability to make judgments and effective decisions about patient care. Formal education aside, in order to realize the goal of providing quality, safe, state-of-the-art patient care, nurses need to make a commitment to ongoing education and the incorporation of new knowledge based on evidence.

Nursing Research

Although it is commonly accepted that best practices are based on decisions validated by sound, scientific evidence, the rate at which current research is translated into nursing practice is often slow. Many nurses today are influenced to some extent by what is known as *knowledge creep* (Pape, 2003). This is a term used to describe the slow percolation of research ideas and findings into the minds, and eventually practice, of clinicians (Polit & Beck, 2004). This phenomenon, however, does not include a conscious decision by the clinician to make a change in practice.

Johns Hopkins Nursing fosters an environment that facilitates the practice of research-based, professional nursing. Nursing research uses qualitative and quantitative systematic methods and an EBP approach directed toward the study and improvement of patient care, patient-care systems, and patient outcomes. The organization supplies the infrastructure required to provide excellence in nursing research and evidence-based practice through mentors, skill-building programs, financial support, computer access, and referral to research consultative services. Nursing leadership supports and encourages the utilization and conduct of nursing research to generate new knowledge and inform practice. The use of research and EBP produces better patient outcomes in health-care organizations because patient-care decisions are conscientiously based on the best scientific evidence (Crowther, Maroulis, Shafer-Winter, & Hader, 2002; Melnyk, 1999).

Evidence-Based Practice: The Core

At the core of the JHNEBP Model is evidence. The core is composed of sources of evidence that form the basis for making decisions about nursing practice, education, and research. Research findings are the strongest type of evidence on which decisions about nursing practice should be made. Research, however, answers a specific question under specific conditions, and the outcome may not be readily transferable to another clinical setting or patient population. Before transferring the evidence to individual situations, carefully consider the quality of research, the relevance of its findings to the clinical setting, and whether the benefit to the patient outweighs any adverse effects (McInnes et al., 2001).

In many cases, research relevant to a particular nursing practice question may be unavailable or limited. Consequently, it is important in the decision-making process to examine and evaluate other types of available evidence—such as clinical guidelines, literature reviews, recommendations from national and local professional organizations, regulations, quality improvement data, and program evaluations—along with expert opinion, patient experience, and clinician judgment and expertise.

Incorporating patient preferences into clinical decision making is becoming more prevalent (McInnes et al., 2001). A patient's values, beliefs, and preferences may influence the patient's desire to comply with treatments despite best evidence. Skills are required by the clinician to maintain a balanced view that not only allows the patient to be involved in decisions, but also effectively and sensitively conveys to the patient the reason why a particular treatment is recommended (McInnes et al., 2001).

Internal and External Factors

The JHNEBP Model is depicted as an open system that is comprised of interrelated components. As an open system, the outputs from this model (decisions about practice, education, and research) are influenced by internal and external factors. *External factors* may include accreditation bodies, legislation, quality measures, regulations, and standards. Accreditation (e.g., the Joint Commission, Commission on Accreditation of Rehabilitation Facilities) requires an organization to achieve and maintain high standards of practice and quality. Legislative (local, state, and federal) and regulatory bodies enact laws and regulations that are designed to protect the public and promote access to health-care services. Failure to follow these laws and regulations may have adverse effects on an organization, most often financial. Examples of regulatory agencies include the Center for Medicare and Medicaid Services, Food and Drug Administration, and state boards of nursing. State nursing boards regulate nursing practice and enforce the Nurse Practice Act, which also serves to protect the public. Quality measures (outcome and performance data) and professional standards serve as yardsticks for evaluating current practice and identifying areas of needed improvement or change. Additionally, there are many external stakeholders—such as the community, media, special interest groups, and third party payors—that exert varying degrees of influence on the organization (Longest, Rakich, & Darr, 2000). Despite the diversity among these external factors, one prevalent trend is the expectation that organizations base their health-care practices and standards on sound evidence.

Internal factors may include organizational culture (values and beliefs), environment (leadership support, resource allocations, patient services, organizational mission, organizational priorities, availability of technology, library support, finance, and so on), equipment and supplies, staffing, and standards (the organization's own policies, procedures, and protocols). Enacting EBP within an organization requires (1) a culture that believes EBP will lead to optimal patient outcomes, (2) strong leadership support at all levels with the necessary resource allocation (human, technological, and financial) to sustain the process, and (3) establishing clear expectations by incorporating EBP into standards and job descriptions. Knowledge and an evaluation of the patient population, the health-care organization, and the internal and external factors are essential components for the successful implementation and perpetuation of EBP within an organization.

The JHNEBP Process: Practice Question, Evidence, and Translation

The JHNEBP process can be simply described as Practice question, Evidence, and Translation (PET), which is shown in Appendix D. The process of translating evidence into practice begins with the identification of a *practice question*, issue, or concern. This is one of the most crucial steps, because how the question is posed drives the remaining steps in the process. After the question is determined, a search for *evidence* is conducted. The evidence is then synthesized and appraised. Based on this appraisal, a determination is made as to whether the evidence supports a change or improvement in practice.

If indeed the evidence supports a change in practice, then evidence *translation* occurs—the practice change is planned for and implemented. The change is then evaluated to see if the desired outcomes were obtained. The final step in translation is the dissemination of the results to patients, staff, hospital stakeholders, and, if appropriate, the local and national community.

Practice Question

The first phase of the process is the development of an answerable EBP question. The question is identified and refined, the scope of the question is determined, and an interdisciplinary team is formed. The following steps are included in the Project Management Tool (Appendix E):

Step 1: Identify an EBP question

The clinical, educational, or administrative EBP question is identified. Keeping the question narrow and specific will make the search for evidence more manageable and will also help guide the search. For example, the question "What is the best way to stop the transmission of methicillin-resistant staphylococcus aureus (MRSA)?" is extremely broad and could encompass many interventions and all practice settings. In contrast, a more focused question is, "What are the best environmental strategies for preventing the spread of MRSA in adult critical care units?" This narrows the question to environmental interventions, such as room cleaning; limits the age group to adults; and limits the practice setting to critical care. The PET process uses the PICO approach (Sackett, Straus, Richardson, Rosenberg, & Haynes, 2000), which narrows the question by identifying the following:

- <u>P</u>atient, population, or problem

- <u>I</u>ntervention

- <u>C</u>omparison with other treatments

- <u>O</u>utcomes

The Question Development Tool (Appendix A) guides the team in defining the issue, how and why it was identified, the scope of the issue, and the PICO format. The tool also assists with looking for evidence and choosing a search strategy. Refer to Chapter 4 for more details regarding the development of an answerable EBP practice question.

Step 2: Define the scope of the practice question

The problem or question may relate to the care of an individual patient, a specific population of patients, or the general patient population in the organization. Defining the scope of the problem assists the team in identifying the appropriate individuals and stakeholders who should be involved in, and kept informed of, the EBP process.

Step 3: Assign responsibility for leadership

For the EBP process to be successful, a leader responsible for facilitating the process and for keeping it moving forward must be identified. If possible, the leader should be experienced in evidence-based practice and have the necessary communication skills to work with an interdisciplinary team. It is also helpful for this individual to be knowledgeable of the organizational structure and strategies for implementing change within the organization.

Step 4: Recruit an interdisciplinary team

When recruiting an interdisciplinary team, it is important to include team members for whom the question holds relevance. When team members are interested and invested in addressing a specific practice question, the work of the team is generally more effective. It is recommended that individuals such as bedside clinicians, who are close to the problem and issues, be included. Additionally, consider including relevant stakeholders, such as clinical specialists, committee members (e.g., Research, Standards of Care and Practice, or Quality Improvement committees), physicians, dietitians, pharmacists, and occupational and physical therapists. To make the group more manageable, attempts should be made to keep the group small, i.e., 6–8 individuals.

Step 5: Schedule a team conference

Setting up the first EBP team conference can be a challenge and includes such activities as (1) reserving a room conducive to group discussion with adequate space; (2) asking team members to bring their calendars so that subsequent meetings can be scheduled; (3) ensuring that a team member is assigned to record discussion points and group decisions, and to keep track of important items (e.g., copies of the EBP tools, extra paper, dry erase board, and so on); (4) providing for a place to keep project files; and (5) establishing a time line for the process.

Evidence

The second phase of the PET process deals with the search for, and appraisal of, the best available evidence. Based on the results of this appraisal, recommendations are made by the team regarding needed practice changes.

Step 6: Conduct an internal and external search for evidence

Team members determine the type of evidence to search for and who will be responsible for conducting the search and bringing the items back to the committee for review. Enlisting the help of a health information specialist (library support) is critical. This will save time and help to ensure a comprehensive search. Refer to Chapters 6 and 7 for a detailed discussion of research and non-research evidence and their appraisal. Some examples of evidence are listed below:

- Research studies

- EBP practice guidelines

- Quality improvement data

- Position statements from professional organizations

- Opinions of internal and external experts

- Regulatory, safety, or risk management data

- Community standards

- Patient surveys and satisfaction data

Step 7: Appraise all types of evidence

Research and non-research evidence are appraised for their strength and quality. The Research Evidence Appraisal (Appendix F) and the Non-Research Evidence Appraisal (Appendix G) assist the team in this activity. The front of each tool includes a set of key questions to determine the type of evidence, its strength, and its quality. The back of each tool includes reference definitions for each evidence type and a scale to rate the evidence quality. The PET process uses a I–V scale to determine the strength of the evidence, with I the strongest and V the weakest (Appendix B). A second scale for quality includes criteria that allows the team to rate the quality of each piece of evidence as high, good, or low/major flaw. The team reviews each item of evidence, and consensus determines both the strength and quality. The Individual Evidence Summary (Appendix H) tracks the team's decisions about each piece of evidence.

Step 8: Summarize the evidence

The team totals the amount of evidence for each level using the Overall Evidence Summary (Appendix I). Then the findings for each level (I–V) are summarized in narrative form, and the overall quality for each level is determined by team consensus.

Step 9: Rate the strength of the evidence

The team makes a determination as to the overall strength and quality of the body of evidence that they have appraised. Refer to Chapters 6 and 7 for a detailed discussion on determining the overall evidence.

Step 10: Develop recommendations for change in systems or processes of care based on the strength of the evidence

Based on the overall appraisal of the evidence strength and quality, the team develops recommendations related to the practice question. For example, if the best available evidence includes good to high quality experimental or quasi-experimental studies, then a sound basis for making a practice change exists. However, if the overall evidence is primarily non-research, i.e., expert opinion, clinical guidelines, and quality improvement data, changes should be made cautiously. Risks and benefits of making the change should be carefully considered. Initiating a change as a pilot study (with a limited set of patients) to determine if the change is effective and whether there are any unanticipated adverse effects is strongly recommended.

Translation

In the third phase of the process, the EBP team determines if the changes to practice are feasible given the target setting. If so, an action plan is created. The change is then implemented and evaluated and the results are communicated to appropriate individuals both internal and external to the organization.

Step 11: Determine the appropriateness and feasibility of translating recommendations into the specific practice setting

The team communicates and obtains feedback from appropriate organizational leadership, bedside clinicians, and all other stakeholders affected by the practice change to determine if the change is appropriate and feasible for the specific practice setting. It is also essential to obtain organizational support, which helps ensure that necessary resources are allocated to make the change.

Step 12: Create an action plan

The team develops a plan to implement the recommended practice change, which may include (1) the development of (or change to) a protocol, guideline, critical pathway, or system/process related to the EBP question, (2) the development of a detailed time line assigning team members to the tasks needed to implement the change (including the evaluation process and reporting of results), and (3) the solicitation of feedback from organizational leadership, bedside clinicians, and other stakeholders on the action plan.

Step 13: Implement the change

Implementation begins. When implementing a change, it is important to ensure that all stakeholders are educated on the practice change, the implementation plan, and the process for evaluating the practice change. This may include verbal and written communication. EBP team members should be available to answer any questions and to troubleshoot problems that may arise during the implementation.

Step 14: Evaluate outcomes

The team evaluates the degree to which the identified outcomes were met. Although positive outcomes are desired, unexpected outcomes often provide opportunities for learning. When unexpected outcomes occur, the team should examine why these outcomes occurred. This examination may indicate the need to make alterations to the practice change or in the implementation process, followed by re-evaluation. Additionally, the evaluation of change should be incorporated into the organization's quality improvement (QI) process so that there is a time line for measurement, evaluation, and reporting of follow-up action.

Step 15: Report the results of the preliminary evaluation to decision makers

When the evaluation is complete, the team again reports the results to appropriate organizational leadership, bedside clinicians, and all other stakeholders. Even if the results are unfavorable, it is important to share the findings. Sharing the results, whether negative or positive, helps to disseminate new knowledge and the generation of additional practice or research questions.

Step 16: Secure support from decision makers to implement the recommended change internally

If the evaluation of the results of the pilot is favorable, the team then obtains organizational support (human, material, and financial) to implement the change fully throughout the organization.

Step 17: Identify the next steps

EBP team members review the process and findings and consider if there are any lessons that should be shared or additional steps to be taken. These may include a new question that has emerged from the process, the need to do more research on the topic, additional training that may be required, suggestions for new tools, writing an article on the process or outcome, or preparing for an oral or poster presentation at a professional conference. There may be other problems identified that have no evidence base, requiring the development of a research protocol.

Step 18: Communicate the findings

This final step of the process is often overlooked and requires strong organizational support. As mentioned above, the results of the EBP project, at a minimum, need to be communicated to the organization. However, depending on the scope of the EBP question and the outcome, serious consideration should be given to the communication of findings external to the organization in appropriate professional journals or through presentations at national organizations.

Summary

This chapter introduces the JHNEBP Model and the steps of the PET process. Nursing staff members from a variety of academic backgrounds have successfully used this process with mentorship and organizational support. Nurses have found it very rewarding to use this process—both to understand the basis for their current nursing interventions and to incorporate changes into their practice based on evidence (Newhouse, Dearholt, Poe, Pugh, & White, 2005).

References

American Nurses Association. (2004). *Nursing scope and standards of practice.* Washington, DC: Author.

Crowther, M., Maroulis, A., Shafer-Winter, N., & Hader, R. (2002). Evidence-based development of a hospital-based heart failure center. *Online Journal of Knowledge Synthesis for Nursing, e9* (1), 123-127. Retrieved October 19, 2007, from http://www.blackwell-synergy.com/toc/wvn/e9/1

Longest, B. B., Jr., Rakich, J., & Darr, K. (2000). *Managing health services organizations and systems* (4th ed.; pp. 27-28). Baltimore, MD: Health Professions Press.

McInnes, E., Harvey, G., Duff. L., Fennessy, G., Seers, K. & Clark, E. (2001). Implementing evidence-based practice in clinical situations. *Nursing Standard, 15*(41), 40-44.

Melnyk, B. M. (1999). Building a case for evidence-based practice: Inhalers vs. nebulizers. *Pediatric Nursing, 25*(1), 101-103.

Newhouse, R., Dearholt, S., Poe, S., Pugh, L., & White, L. (2005). Evidence-based practice. *Journal of Nursing Administration, 35*(1), 35-40.

Pape, T. M. (2003). Evidence-based nursing practice: To infinity and beyond. *The Journal of Continuing Education in Nursing, 34*(4), 154-190.

Polit, D., & Beck, C. T. (2004). *Nursing research: Principles and methods* (7th ed.). Baltimore, MD: Lippincott Williams & Wilkins.

Porter-O'Grady, T. (1984). *Shared governance for nursing: A creative approach to professional accountability.* Rockville, MD: Aspen Systems Corporation.

Sackett, D. L., Straus, S. E., Richardson, W. S., Rosenberg, W., & Haynes, R. B. (2000). *Evidence based medicine: How to practice and teach EBM.* Edinburgh, Scotland: Churchill.

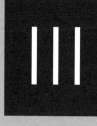

Practice, Evidence, Translation (PET)

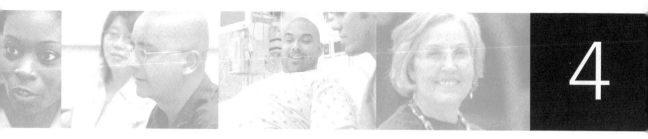

4

The Practice Question

Practice questions proliferate for clinical, administrative, and education nurses charged with making sound, evidence-based decisions. Answers to questions are occasionally available through evidence summaries, such as systematic reviews, integrative reviews, literature reviews, or guidelines available in print or electronic media. More often, however, a synthesis is not available for many nursing questions. This chapter discusses the first phase of the evidence-based practice (EBP) process, asking a practice question, and

- explores the origin of practice problems appropriate for an EBP approach

- proposes criteria for the selection of a practice problem

- describes how to use the PICO framework to create an answerable EBP question

- identifies the steps in forming an EBP team

The EBP process known as PET conceptualizes asking a practice question, finding evidence, and translating the evidence into practice. Within the PET process, the practice question phase includes five operational steps. The first step is to identify the practice problem. It is extremely important to generate and refine the question, because all subsequent actions and decisions build on the problem definition. The JHNEBP Question Development Tool (Appendix A) can facilitate the first phase.

The Origin of Practice Problems

Health-care team members have many opportunities to identify clinical problems, educational concerns, and administrative issues surrounding their areas of practice. An EBP approach is appropriate to inform and guide decisions in any of these areas.

The process of forming an EBP question often begins when one of the following questions arises:

1. What evidence is the basis for this treatment?

2. Is there a scientific basis for this treatment?

3. What was the rationale for making that decision?

4. What are the clinical implications of this practice?

5. Why are we doing this, and why are we doing it this way?

6. Is there a way to do this better, more efficiently, and more cost-effectively?

7. Does this involve any time-wasting activities?

8. Are these the best achievable outcomes?

Developing an answerable question, the first step in the EBP process, addresses a clinical, administrative, or educational problem. The problem can emerge from multiple sources (See Table 4.1).

Table 4.1.   Sources of Evidence-Based Practice Problems

Safety/risk management concerns

Unsatisfactory patient outcomes

Wide variations in practice

Significant financial concerns

Differences between hospital and community practice

Clinical practice issue is a concern

Procedure or process is a time waster

Clinical practice issue has no scientific base

Sources of nursing problems include problem-focused triggers or knowledge-focused triggers (Titler et al., 1994; Titler et al., 2001). *Problem-focused triggers* include risk management data, quality improvement results, variances in benchmarking or financial data, and recognition of clinical problems. *Knowledge-focused triggers* include new sources of evidence, changes in standards or guidelines, philosophies of care, and new information provided by the organizational standards committees.

Problems may be a recurring or priority issue within an organization, or a practice that has no benefit and is questioned by a nurse's expertise and experience. For example, clinical questions may relate to why one patient population has better outcomes than another does. There may be a difference in practice among nurses, nursing units, or peers outside of the organization. The potential for problems to generate practice questions is limitless. Problems are significant for evidence-based practice projects when results lead to improvements in patient health, organization of systems, or education. This point is worthy of further discussion, because not all problems should be approached using the PET methodology.

The JHNEBP Question Development Tool (Appendix A) can be used to create a practice question. Begin with a clear statement of the problem or issue. Define the practice area (clinical, administrative, or education). Next, define the origin of the problem (check boxes are provided) and the scope of the problem (individual, population, or system/organization). Answering these questions will help to assess the problem's significance, size, and scope to evaluate the appropriateness of an EBP approach.

Criteria for Selecting EBP Projects

Evidence-based practice requires time, availability of evidence, EBP skills, and leadership support. Consequently, using the EBP model and process may not be practical for all questions. Choose questions that have a high return on quality and cost-efficient care. Before embarking on a project, and committing the time and resources necessary for the EBP process, consider the following questions: Would the practice changes resulting from this project improve clinical outcomes, unit processes, or patient or nurse satisfaction? Would they reduce the cost of care and be implementable, given the current infrastructure? If the problem is important and the solution has potential to improve the quality of care, then generate a question to focus the project.

The Background and Foreground Question

There are two main EBP question types—background and foreground (Sackett, Rosenberg, Gray, Haynes, & Richardson, 1996; Sackett, Straus, Richardson, Rosenberg, & Haynes, 2000). A *background question* is a general, best practice question that is broad and produces a wide range of evidence for review: What are the best nursing interventions to manage pain for patients with a history of substance abuse? This question would produce evidence related to pharmacology, alternative therapies, behavioral contracting, and biases in prescribing and administering pain medication. Background evidence can provide the state of the science about a problem and can lead to a refined foreground question.

A *foreground question* is a focused question that includes specific comparisons: Is behavioral contracting or mutual goal setting more effective in improving the pain experience for patients with a history of substance abuse? Foreground questions produce a very refined, limited body of evidence specific to the EBP question.

When asking a background question, the evidence review can become complex. It is helpful to organize the EBP project by breaking down the components of the problem into the appropriate number of foreground questions. Create questions that relate to each of the components identified. For example, if the problem requires identification of best practices in falls prevention, questions might address risk as-sessment and a variety of interventions. After the importance of the EBP project is established and the general problem identified, the next step is to refine the question.

Developing an Answerable EBP Question

The thoughtful development of a well-structured EBP question is important, be-cause the question drives the strategies used to search for evidence. Making the EBP question as specific as possible helps to identify and narrow search terms. This reduc-es the time spent searching for relevant evidence and increases the likelihood of find-ing it. Making the EBP question as specific as possible helps to focus the EBP project and provide a sensitive evidence review that is specific to the problem and question. It also helps in clearly communicating the target population (age, gender, ethnicity, diagnosis, procedure, etc.), so that the translation of the recommendations is planned appropriately. Chapter 5 describes using key words for evidence searching.

To construct an answerable EBP question that promotes an efficient search for evidence, the PICO (described below) format is helpful (Richardson, Wilson, Nishi-kawa, & Hayward, 1995). PICO frames the problem clearly and facilitates the evi-dence search by identifying core key words.

P – Patient, population, or problem. Identify the type of patient, the population, or the problem succinctly. Consider attributes such as age, gender, patient setting, and symptoms. For example, the patients of interest may be adult surgical inpatients between the ages of 20 and 50 years old with a peripheral intravenous catheter (IV).

I – Intervention. The intervention can be a treatment or a clinical, educational, or administrative intervention. For example, the intervention may include a process of care, nursing treatments, strategies for education, or assessment approaches. An example of a nursing treatment intervention is the use of saline flushes for peripheral IV maintenance.

C – Comparison with other intervention(s). Identify if a comparison group exists. Will the intervention be compared to another intervention? Not all questions have comparisons, or comparisons may not be readily apparent. For example, the com-parison may be the use of heparin (vs. saline) flushes for peripheral IV maintenance.

O – Outcomes. Identify the outcomes of interest. Outcomes may include quality of life, improved treatment outcomes, decreased rate of adverse events, improved patient safety, decreased cost, or improved patient satisfaction. For example, an outcome of interest may be improvement in IV patency over a specified time or a decrease in the incidence of phlebitis.

This example uses PICO to create a foreground question: For adult surgical inpatients between the ages of 20 and 50 with a peripheral intravenous catheter, does the use of saline to flush the peripheral IV maintain IV patency and decrease phlebitis over 48 hours when compared to heparin flushes?

The EBP Team

After a question is clearly stated in PICO format, the next step is to assemble the team. Consider the scope of the EBP question when assembling the team. The scope of the problem may be at the individual patient, population, or organizational level. Depending on the scope of the question, different team members should be included. For example, if the problem is postoperative hypothermia management, anesthesia and surgery representatives should be included. Anticipation of how the recommendations of the project will be implemented, and whose practice they will affect, determines which individuals or groups should be involved. The JHNEBP Project Management Tool (Appendix E) can guide the process.

After the team is assembled, leadership selection can occur. The team should designate a leader who possesses skills in leading a meeting and keeping a project on track. The leader must be able to articulate the team's recommendations and influence implementation.

An EBP team must consist of members who have expertise with the problem. Often, this means an interdisciplinary team, including nurses, physicians, and other professional staff who contribute significantly to care of the patient population selected. For example, if the question relates to best practices in the management of nausea for the patient undergoing chemotherapy, the team may consist of nurses, pharmacists, and oncologists. Keep the team size small and efficient. Team members will need to commit to attending the meetings, completing their evidence review prior to the meeting, presenting their evidence, participating in the practice recommendation, and being responsible for the team's decisions. The number of people should be small enough to promote efficiency of the process and large enough to provide content expertise. If team members have never conducted an EBP project, they will also need an experienced mentor to help them through the process the first time.

If a background question is posed, consider multiple EBP teams to enable each team to address a specific foreground question, if indicated. This will engage more staff in the process and allow teams to narrow the focus and review smaller bodies of evidence. Each team will then provide a recommendation to its targeted question. If one team focuses on a background question, the body of evidence is far more diverse and the quantity of evidence greater.

The leader schedules the first team conference, with subsequent meetings established so that team members can reserve the time. This is sometimes the most challenging portion of planning the EBP project. Setting a time when the team is available away from the demands of the clinical area within a time line that is practical to complete the project is essential. Team members that work multiple shifts, various days, and in different roles can rarely agree on a time and date without as much as two months' notice. Occasionally, teams with a regularly scheduled meeting established for quality improvement, policy and procedure committee, or other professional responsibilities use the standard meeting time for the EBP project.

Each team member will have different availability and the meetings will need to consider each member's schedule. Some teams schedule a preliminary meeting to refine the practice question, then one or two 8-hour days to review the evidence and make a recommendation. Others have approached scheduling challenges by scheduling 4-hour blocks monthly, or 2-hour meetings every 2 weeks. If multiple meetings will be held, schedule meetings weekly or every 2 weeks, if possible, to keep the team moving forward. Delay between group meetings negatively affects the team's momentum. With the problem identified and refined, and the leader and team selected, the project is ready to move into the evidence phase.

Summary

This chapter introduces the multiple origins of practice problems appropriate for an EBP approach. It is essential to approach this first stage of the EBP project, the practice question, thoughtfully. A well-framed question and appropriate team composition that can complete the process successfully is the ultimate goal. Careful construction of the question and selection of the team will increase the team's efficiency in the EBP process and outcome. A well-formulated practice question guides the generation of key words for the evidence step.

References

American Nurses Association. (2004). *Nursing scope and standards of practice.* Washington, DC: Author.

Crowther, M., Maroulis, A., Shafer-Winter, N., & Hader, R. (2002). Evidence-based development of a hospital-based heart failure center. *Online Journal of Knowledge Synthesis for Nursing, e9*(1), 123-127. Retrieved October 19, 2007, from http://www.blackwell-synergy.com/toc/wvn/e9/1

Longest, B. B., Jr., Rakich, J., & Darr, K. (2000). *Managing health services organizations and systems* (4th ed.; pp. 27-28). Baltimore, MD: Health Professions Press.

McInnes, E., Harvey, G., Duff. L., Fennessy, G., Seers, K. & Clark, E. (2001). Implementing evidence-based practice in clinical situations. *Nursing Standard, 15*(41), 40-44.

Melnyk, B. M. (1999). Building a case for evidence-based practice: Inhalers vs. nebulizers. *Pediatric Nursing, 25*(1), 101-103.

Newhouse, R., Dearholt, S., Poe, S., Pugh, L., & White, L. (2005). Evidence-based practice. *Journal of Nursing Administration, 35*(1), 35-40.

Pape, T. M. (2003). Evidence-based nursing practice: To infinity and beyond. *The Journal of Continuing Education in Nursing, 34*(4), 154-190.

Polit, D., & Beck, C. T. (2004). *Nursing research: Principles and methods* (7th ed.). Baltimore, MD: Lippincott Williams & Wilkins.

Porter-O'Grady, T. (1984). *Shared governance for nursing: A creative approach to professional accountability.* Rockville, MD: Aspen Systems Corporation.

Sackett, D. L., Straus, S. E., Richardson, W. S., Rosenberg, W., & Haynes, R. B. (2000). *Evidence based medicine: How to practice and teach EBM.* Edinburgh, Scotland: Churchill.

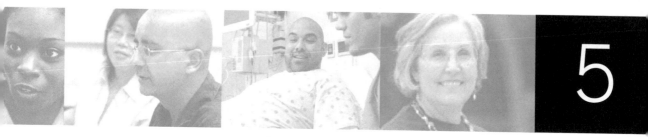

Searching for Evidence

5

Evidence-based practice "requires an emphasis on systematic observation and experience and a reliance on the research literature to substantiate nursing decisions" (Kessenich, Guyatt, & DiCenso, 1997, p. 25). Developing information literacy skills involves being aware of the nursing literature and acquiring the skills to locate and retrieve it. Studies have shown that positive changes in a nurse's information-literacy skills, and confidence in those skills, have a direct impact on nurses' appreciation and application of research. These skills are vital for effective lifelong learning and are a prerequisite to evidence-based practice (Shorten, Wallace, & Crookes, 2001).

Evidence can be collected from a variety of sources, including the Web and proprietary databases. The information explosion has made it difficult for health-care workers, researchers, educators, and policy makers to process all the relevant literature available to them on a daily basis. Evidence-based clinical resources make searching for medical information much easier and faster than in years past. This chapter discusses strategies for evidence searches and

- describes key information formats

- identifies steps in working with an answerable question

- suggests information and evidence resources

- provides tips for search strategies and evaluation of search results

Key Information Formats

Resources to support evidence-based nursing are rapidly evolving (Collins, Voth, DiCenso, & Guyatt, 2005). Those that are preprocessed can be the most practical source of current and reliable information for front-line staff nurses. *Preprocessed resources* are materials that have been reviewed and chosen based on methodological standards for inclusion. Identifying these resources involves knowing the format of the information needed to help answer the practice question. Literature searching is a key feature of the EBP process, as it helps nurses to enrich their clinical practice and experience by locating up-to-date evidence important to the care they deliver. Evidence comes from many sources, such as primary evidence, evidence summaries, and translation literature.

Primary evidence is usually data collected at the point of patient contact. This evidence can come from hospital-wide data, clinical trials, peer-reviewed research journals, conference reports, monographs, or summaries of information from data sets, such as the Center for Medicare and Medicaid Services' Minimum Data Set. A few examples of databases used to find this type of information are MEDLINE, CINAHL, institutional repositories, and library catalogs.

Evidence summaries come from synthesized literature and provide broader foci on topics. They are usually found in systematic reviews, integrative reviews, book chapters, and meta-analyses. Databases for these resources include library catalogs, online book collections, MEDLINE, The Cochrane Library, MD Consult, and UpTo-Date. Quality improvement and financial information from a topic-specific database, such as Health Business FullText, can provide valuable cost and quality information for hospital administrators and case managers.

Translation literature includes quality-filtered Internet and Intranet sources. This literature can come from practice guidelines, critical pathways, care plans, clinical innovations, protocols, standards, and evidence-based practice centers, as well as peer-reviewed journals and bibliographic research databases.

The Answerable Question

After the information needed for a practice problem is identified and converted into an answerable question (see Chapter 4), the search for evidence begins and includes the following steps:

1. Selecting searchable keywords, synonyms, and related terms from the answerable question

2. Identifying the best sources to find preprocessed information and choosing appropriate search tools

3. Developing search strategies and performing the search using controlled vocabularies, limits, and Boolean operators

4. Evaluating the result set for validity and authority

5. Recording search strategy and saving results

EBP Search Examples

Selecting possible keywords and synonyms from the clinical question should be the first step in finding the evidence. Appendix A is the JHNEBP Question Development Tool, which includes keywords based on the question raised in PICO format. A search template can help break down the answerable question into keywords.

Consider the following answerable question: What is the effect of nursing care on the prevention of pressure ulcers for elderly men with hip fractures? The terms *nursing care*, *pressure ulcers*, and *elderly* may be in an initial query. Table 5.1 illustrates the use of the PICO format to find these terms. However, consider additional related terms such as *aged*, *patient care planning*, *decubitus ulcer*, *wound*, and *management* for the search.

Table 5.1.   PICO Example

P = Patient with a fractured hip

I = Best nursing interventions

C = Not applicable

O = Prevent pressure ulcers

It is also useful to remember the context of the problem when thinking of similar terms. For example, the standardized nursing diagnosis of acute pain and its outcomes can be described as: *disruptive effects of pain, psychological responses to pain*, etc. These outcomes are diagnosis specific, not based on interventions.

Box 5.1 demonstrates the development of an answerable question and search strategy from specific situations.

Box 5.1

Example: Zinc for children?

You are a school nurse who regularly visits a number of elementary and middle schools (children ages 5 to 13 years) in your region. It is cold and flu season once again. One of the teachers stops you in the hall to ask you a question about his 10-year-old daughter, who has a cold. He has heard that zinc lozenges can help to relieve cold symptoms and is wondering if they really do work and whether it is okay to give them to children.

PICO:

Patient (children with colds). **Intervention** (zinc lozenges). **Comparable Intervention** (other treatments or no treatment). **Outcome** (relief of symptoms).

Answerable question:

In children with colds, are zinc lozenges safe and effective for relief of cold symptoms?

Initial search terms:	**Related terms:**
Zinc	Lozenges, zinc acetate, zinc gluconate
Child	Common cold, rhinovirus
Cold	Children, youth

Example: A new prescription?

Your next patient is a 72-year-old woman with osteoarthritis of the knees and moderate hypertension, accompanied by her daughter, a lab tech from the hospital. The daughter wants you to give her mother a prescription for one of the COX-2 inhibitors. She has heard that they cause less GI bleeding. Her mother is concerned that the new drugs will mean more out-of-pocket costs each month.

PICO:

Patient (72-year-old woman with osteoarthritis of the knee and moderate hypertension). **Intervention** (COX-2 Inhibitor). **Comparable Intervention** (other NSAIDs). **Outcome** (less GI bleeding, pain relief).

Answerable question:

In a 72-year-old-woman with osteoarthritis of the knee, can COX-2 Inhibitor use decrease the risk of GI bleeding compared with other NSAIDs?

Initial search terms:	**Related terms:**
COX-2 Inhibitors	NSAIDs, aspirin, ibuprofen
Osteoarthritis	Arthritis, therapy
GI bleeding	Gastrointestinal bleeding, stomach ulcers
Elderly	Side effects, adverse effects
	Aged, female

Controlled Vocabularies

Controlled vocabularies, such as taxonomies, classification systems, or nomenclature, are specific terms used to identify concepts within an index or database. The Dewey Decimal System is probably the most well-known controlled vocabulary. Specifically, controlled vocabularies are official indexing terms used by the organizers of a database to describe each concept so that all the items on the same topic have the same subject heading. They mandate the use of predefined, authorized terms that have been preselected by the designer of the controlled vocabulary—as opposed to natural language vocabularies where there is no restriction on the vocabulary used. Controlled vocabularies are important tools, because they allow the database query to gather citations with concepts relevant to the topic but not exactly what was entered. They ensure consistency and reduce ambiguity inherent in human languages where the same concept may have different names. Additionally, they often improve the accuracy of free text searching by reducing irrelevant items in the retrieval list. A good example is the term *football*, which can be ambiguous with soccer, rugby, or American football depending on geographic location.

Some well known vocabularies are:

- PubMed (MEDLINE) = MeSH (Medical Subject Headings)

- CINAHL = CINAHL Subject Headings

- PsycINFO = Thesaurus of Psychological Index Terms

- Nursing Interventions Classification (NIC)

- Nursing Outcomes Classification (NOC)

Nursing-specific controlled vocabularies, such as NANDA International Taxonomy and CINAHL Subject Headings, should be consulted to retrieve nursing-specific information. However, not all controlled vocabularies are created equal. It has been suggested that differences between the terminologies of medicine and nursing can impede the efficient retrieval of evidence-based nursing literature (Lavin et al., 2002). For example, the phrase *patient monitoring* from CINAHL Subject Headings translates into *physiologic monitoring* in Medical Subject Headings (MeSH). Another good example is the term *nursing shortage*, used to describe the decline in the nursing workforce. In PubMed, articles relevant to this topic are found when combining the MeSH terms *health manpower* and *hospital nursing staff* or when qualifying the MeSH term *nursing* with the subheading of *manpower*. The CINAHL Subject heading for *nursing shortage* is *nursing shortage*. Additionally, there are subject headings related to evidence-based practice in regard to the publication type, such as *experimental studies, meta-analysis, controlled trials, quasi-experimental studies, community studies, qualitative studies*, and so on. Databases that use controlled vocabularies often have a separate search engine for finding them. The MeSH Database in PubMed is one example.

Selecting Information and Evidence Resources

Many information resources are available in electronic formats. Table 5.2 lists useful Web sites.

Table 5.2.   Online Evidence

Online Journal of Clinical Innovations: www.cinahl.com/cexpress/ojcionline3/index.html

The Cochrane Collaboration: www.cochrane.org/index.htm

Cochrane Collaboration Hand Search Manual: www.cochrane.org/resources/hsmpt1.htm

CRISP: Computer Retrieval of Information on Scientific Projects: http://crisp.cit.nih.gov

EBN Online, Evidence Based Nursing: http://ebn.bmj.com

EBSCO Publishing: www.ebscohost.com/thisSubject.php?marketID=2&subjectID=8

Joanna Briggs Institute: www.joannabriggs.edu.au

Journal of Nursing Scholarship: www.nursingsociety.org/publications/JNS_main.html

NANDA International Taxonomy II: www.nanda.org/html/taxonomy.html

NGC—National Guidelines Clearinghouse: www.guideline.gov

PubMed: www.ncbi.nlm.nih.gov/sites/entrez?db=PubMed

PubMed Central Home Page: www.pubmedcentral.nih.gov

Registry of Nursing Research—Virginia Henderson International Nursing Library: www.nursinglibrary.org/portal/main.aspx

TRIP Database: For Evidence Based Medicine (EBM): www.tripdatabase.com/index.html

UpToDate: Putting Clinical Information Into Practice: www.uptodate.com

Worldviews on Evidence Based Nursing: www.blackwellpublishing.com/journal.asp?ref=1545-102X&site=1

CINAHL

The Cumulative Index to Nursing and Allied Health Literature (CINAHL) database covers approximately 2,700 nursing, allied health, biomedical, and consumer health journals, as well as publications of both the American Nurses Association and the National League for Nursing from 1982 to the present. The database is produced by EBSCO Information Systems and offers various options, including CINAHL with Full-Text, CINAHL Plus, and CINAHL Plus with Full-Text, each with various depths of coverage and full-text availability. CINAHL provides references to dissertations, standards of practice, book chapters, legal cases, clinical innovations, critical paths, drug records, research instruments, and clinical trials. CINAHL uses a standard subject-heading vocabulary that includes nursing classifications and evidence-based filters for searching, such as research (for publication types) or evidence-based practice (as a special interest category). Within the search *artificial nails* AND *infection*, the user can select peer-reviewed articles by selecting Refine Search on the search screen (see Figure 5.1).

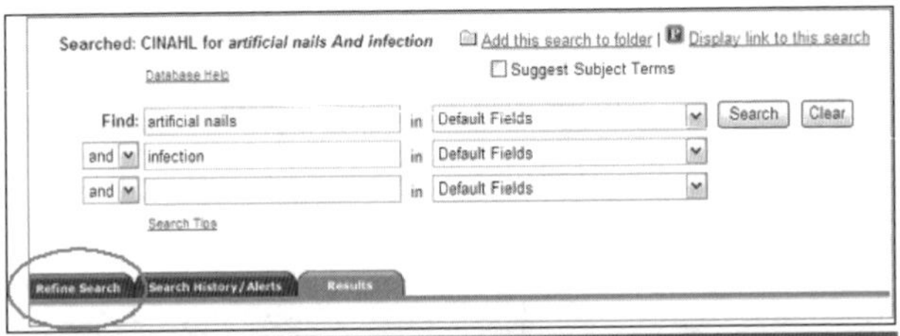

Figure 5.1. Refining the Search.

MEDLINE (PubMed)

The MEDLINE database, available free of charge through PubMed, is provided by the National Library of Medicine and is widely known as the premier source for bibliographic and abstract coverage of biomedical literature. It includes citation information from a variety of indices that reference more than 5,000 journals, at least 300 of which are explicit to nursing. PubMed also contains evidence-based filters in its Clinical Queries search engine (see Figure 5.2). Clinical Queries uses predetermined clinical filters to find relevant information topics relating to one of five clinical study categories: *therapy, diagnosis, etiology, prognosis,* and *clinical prediction guides.* Searches can be *sensitive* (include most relevant articles but probably include some less relevant ones) or *specific* (include mostly relevant articles but probably omit a few). Clinical Queries also includes a search filter for systematic reviews, combining search terms with citations identified as systematic reviews, meta-analyses, reviews of clinical trials, evidence-based medicine, consensus development conferences, and guidelines.

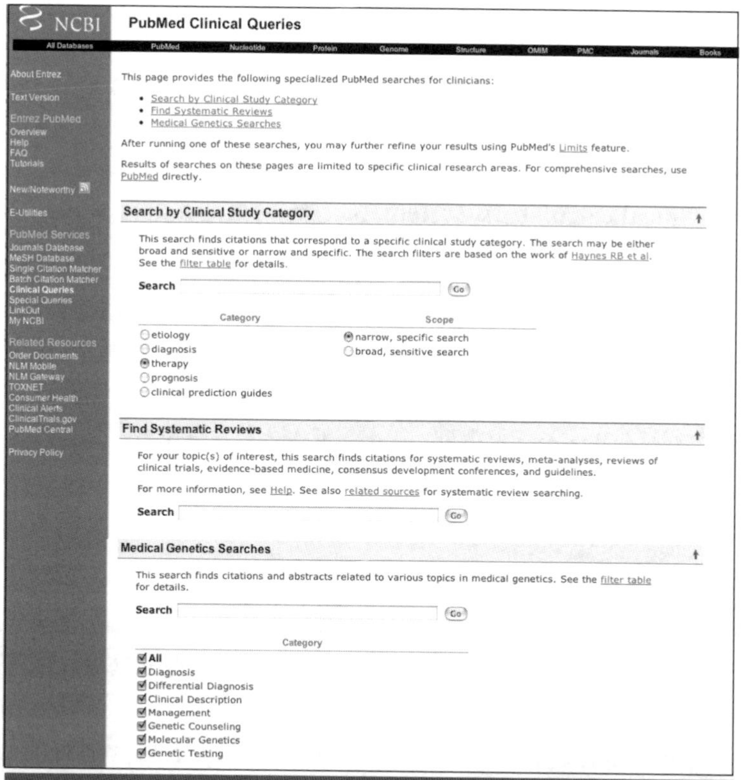

Figure 5.2. Clinical Queries

The Cochrane Library

The Cochrane Library is a collection of seven databases used to locate *evidence summaries*, or synthesized reviews of health-care interventions, including the Cochrane Database of Systematic Reviews. The reviews are highly structured and systematic, including or excluding evidence based on explicit quality criteria, to minimize bias. Cochrane Reviews are based on the best available information about health-care interventions. They explore the evidence for and against the effectiveness and appropriateness of treatments (medications, surgery, education, etc.) in specific circumstances. Cochrane reviews address clearly formulated questions: Does fluoride help prevent tooth decay in children? Can antibiotics help in alleviating the symptoms of a sore throat? Abstracts of reviews are available free of charge from the Cochrane Web site; however, full reviews are available by subscription. The Cochrane Library can be a solid source for locating evidence-based interventions in nursing practice.

Other Resources and Strategies

The Turning Research into Practice Database (TRIP) is a meta-search engine for evidence-based health-care topics. It peruses hundreds of evidence-based medicine and evidence-based nursing Web sites that contain synopses, clinical answers, textbook information, clinical calculators, systematic reviews, and guidelines. Its filtering system for result retrieval quickly enables it to find information on practice questions.

Another search engine worth mentioning is the Computer Retrieval of Information on Scientific Projects Database (CRISP), which is a United States Government database of federally funded biomedical research projects conducted at universities, hospitals, and other research institutions. Users, including the public, can use CRISP to search for scientific concepts and emerging trends and techniques, or to identify specific projects and/or investigators. It is a good tool for finding experts in a field or similar nursing research questions.

In addition to using bibliographic and Web databases, researchers should also consider hand searching appropriate peer-reviewed journals, which should be evaluated for their methodology and clinical reference. It is estimated that anywhere from 10–15% of articles on a topic will not be found if this step is skipped (Cochrane, 2003). Moreover, systematically searching reference lists and consulting subject specialists and experts in the field can be done.

Although there are many free Web-based resources, some of the quality resources named above have a cost. Many libraries provide access to these resources by paying licensing fees to publishers so their users can access them. When searching these databases and online resources, analyzing the quality and relevance of the studies is up to the user.

The medical librarian is uniquely trained and strategically located to support a nurse's information retrieval. Libraries are an essential gateway to evidence-based information. Medical librarians can offer database and computer skills training in addition to mediated database searching.

There are also journals that provide summaries of literature based on nursing practice, such as the *Online Journal of Clinical Innovations*, and *Worldviews on Evidence-Based Nursing*. *Worldviews* is a new, peer-reviewed journal from Sigma

Theta Tau International that provides knowledge synthesis and research articles on best evidence to support best practices globally for nurses in a wide range of roles, from clinical practice and education to administration and public health-care policy. The *Online Journal of Clinical Innovations,* published by CINAHL Information Systems, provides up-to-date access to research reports, innovation implementation from conferences, and communication with investigators and clinicians. Other journals specific to evidence-based nursing practice include *Evidence-Based Nursing* and *Journal of Nursing Scholarship*.

Web resources can also be consulted, especially if they are from a reputable, authoritative organization whose information is relevant to the practice question. There are many EBP nursing Web sites on the Internet that offer other models of EBP, practice guidelines, and tutorials for additional learning. One such Web site is the Joanna Briggs Institute of the Royal Adelaide Hospital in South Australia. The institute is an international collaboration involving nursing, medical, and allied health researchers, clinicians, academics, and quality managers across 40 countries on every continent. The mission is to facilitate evidence-based health-care practice globally through being a leading international organization for the translation, transfer, and utilization of evidence regarding the feasibility, appropriateness, meaningfulness, and effectiveness of health-care practice. Users should take note of the Best Practice Information Sheets, which are based on systematic reviews of research done at the Institute and around the world.

An additional Internet resource is Sigma Theta Tau International's Virginia Henderson International Nursing Library. The library's Registry of Nursing Research is a database of research studies contributed directly by nurse researchers that provides abstracts of research projects, institutional affiliation of the researcher, contact information, study details, funding sources, and study populations.

The United States government produces The National Guideline Clearinghouse, which is a search engine for finding practice guidelines. This database is available free of charge from the Agency for Healthcare Research and Quality and is a mechanism for obtaining objective, detailed information on clinical practice guidelines from all over the world. The database includes summaries about the guidelines, links to full-text where available, and a guidelines comparison chart.

Tips for Search Strategies and Evaluating Search Results

Search Strategies

After the resource that will help answer the practice question is located, the search begins. Search strategies are developed by breaking the defined question into individual concepts, then selecting words and phrases that describe the concepts. Boolean operators, spelling variations, and limit features can enhance keywords and text. Developing the search strategy to locate information in a database should include the following:

1. Use controlled vocabulary for keywords and phrases. When the correct term is identified, most of the information is grouped together, saving the time of having to search all the other synonyms for that term. Medical Subject Headings in PubMed are searchable in the MeSH Database. Search CINAHL Subject Headings directly in the CINAHL database.

2. Use the Boolean operators AND, OR, and NOT (Figure 5.3). Combine keywords and phrases with controlled vocabulary to produce a promising result set.

3. Because of differences in American and British spelling, think of alternate spellings, such as *tumour* versus *tumor*, *behaviour* versus *behavior*, and *gynaecology* versus *gynecology*. Some databases have mapped the terms together to be synonymous while searching, but many have not.

4. Use limits where appropriate, such as age, date of publication, and language. Search more efficiently by using filters designed to exclude extraneous retrievals. For example, limiting by the research publication type will pull randomized controlled trials or clinical trials into the result set. An initial limit of *English only*, *last 5 years*, and *nursing subset* can greatly reduce the number of citations. In the PubMed example below, an initial search yielded 185 citations. When limited to *last 5 years*, *English only*, and *nursing journals*, the result set dropped to 40 and was more precise (Figure 5.4).

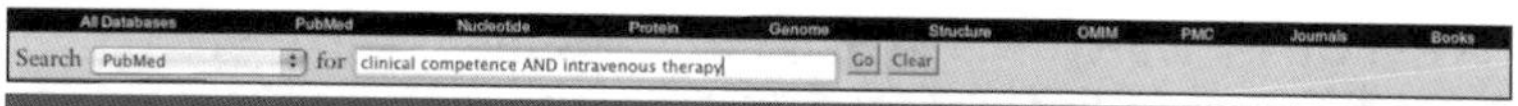

Figure 5.3.   Boolean Operators

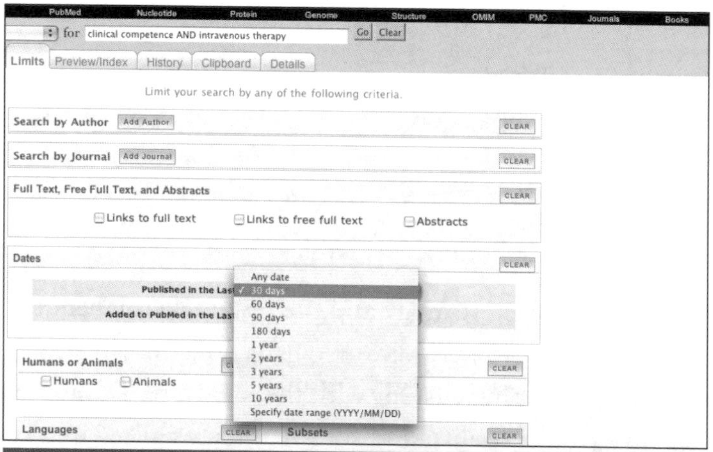

Figure 5.4.   Setting Limits

Reviewing and Evaluating Search Results

The final step in finding the evidence involves reviewing the results to determine whether they are relevant to the EBP question, and then modifying the search strategy if necessary. Each database usually offers a variety of formats and references for review. If a citation meets the needs of the topic, many databases offer a Related Articles or Find More Like This feature to help locate similar articles. If the results are too specific, controlled vocabularies or the Boolean operator OR can broaden the search. If the results are too broad, controlled vocabularies or the Boolean operator AND can narrow the results.

Ask these questions when reviewing search results:

- Who wrote it?

- Who sponsored the research?

- What institutional or organizational affiliation exists?

- When was it published?

- Has it been reviewed? If so, by whom?

- Why was it published?

- Has it been cited? Whom does it cite?

Keep a record of the search strategy and the results. Permanent searches are useful for individuals who want to periodically re-execute a search strategy as the database is updated, thereby keeping current with the literature. Databases will usually allow researchers to save the results, and some databases allow users to save the strategy with it. For those databases that don't provide this function, simply view the strategy within the database and then copy and paste it into a document. Many databases allow researchers to save a strategy within the database and receive update alerts. PubMed does this with MyNCBI (see Figure 5.5). Result sets can also be e-mailed to the user or a colleague, or saved in bibliographic management programs such as EndNote or Reference Manager.

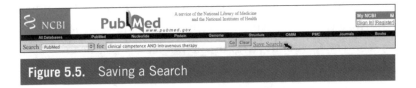

Figure 5.5.   Saving a Search

Compare the results from all the databases and sources of information and then locate full-text articles relevant to answering the evidence-based practice question. Some articles are obtained free of charge from databases such as PubMed Central, but many are subscription-based. Consult with a local health sciences library or public library for information on obtaining articles through interlibrary loan. Assessing the reliability and validity of the research studies selected, or *appraising the evidence*, is the next phase of EBP.

Summary

This chapter not only supports the multi-step evidence-based practice model, it also guides all literature searches. An essential component of evidence-based practice, the literature search is important to any research and publication activity, because it enables researchers to acquire a better understanding of the research topic and an awareness of relevant literature. Information specialists, such as medical librarians, can help with complex search strategies and information retrieval.

Researchers ideally need to use an iterative search process—first examining indexed databases, using keywords in searches, and studying the resulting articles, then refining their searches for optimal retrieval. Keywords, controlled vocabulary, Boolean operators, and limits play an immense role in finding the most relevant material for the practice problem. Currently, alerting services are effective in helping researchers keep up to date with a research topic. Exploring and selecting from the vast array of published information can be a time-consuming task, so it is important to know how to plan and carry out this work effectively.

References

Cochrane Collaboration. (2003). *Cochrane hand search manual.* Retrieved October 22, 2007 from http://www.cochrane.org/resources/hsmpt1.htm

Collins, S., Voth, T., DiCenso, A., & Guyatt, G. (2005). Finding the evidence. In *Evidence-based nursing: A guide to clinical practice.* St. Louis, MO: Elsevier Mosby.

Kessenich, C. R., Guyatt, G. H., & DiCenso, A. (1997). Teaching nursing students evidence-based nursing. *Nurse Educator, 22,* 25-29.

Lavin, M. A., Meyer, G., Krieger, M., McNary, P., Carlson, J., Perry, A. et al. (2002). Essential differences between evidence-based nursing and evidence-based medicine. *International Journal of Nursing Terminologies and Classifications, 13,* 101-106.

Shorten, A., Wallace, M. C., & Crookes, P. A. (2001). Developing information literacy: A key to evidence-based nursing. *International Nursing Review, 48,* 86-92.

Contributing author for this chapter is **Holly A. Willis, MLIS,** director of the McGlannan Library at Mercy Medical Center in Baltimore, Maryland. She earned a BS in biology from Randolph-Macon College in 1995 and obtained her master's in library and information science, specializing in health sciences and medical informatics, from the University of Pittsburgh in 2000. As a liaison librarian with the Welch Medical Library at The Johns Hopkins University, Ms. Willis formed collaborative relationships with 11 academic and clinical departments, including the School of Nursing and the hospital Department of Nursing. As library director at Mercy Medical Center, she oversees all the major functions of the library, including budgeting, policies and procedures, acquisitions, electronic resource management, collection development, outreach, and marketing, as well as library instruction. Ms. Willis is active in medical library organizations and has presented papers at several conferences.

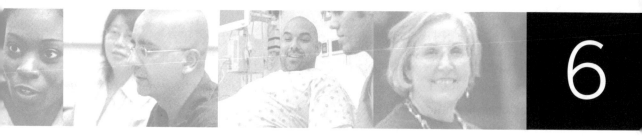

Appraising Research

6

Most evidence-rating schemes recognize that the strongest evidence accumulates from scientific evidence, or research. Within the broad realm of research, many different types of studies exist that vary in terms of the strength of evidence they provide. The current discussion of research evidence addresses the following types of studies: meta-analysis, experimental (randomized controlled trials), quasi-experimental, non-experimental (descriptive and correlational research), meta-synthesis, and qualitative.

This chapter's objectives are to recognize the various types of research evidence as part of an EBP review and to present tips for reading research evidence. The chapter closes with recommendations to clinical nurse leaders to increase the ability of nurses to examine critically their practice through the review and appraisal of scientific evidence.[1]

[1] This book provides basic information about evaluating synthesized evidence from a systematic review. It is important to note that the appraisal of a systematic review has to be considered based upon the highest level of research evidence that the systematic review includes. The reader is cautioned to interpret non-peer reviewed synthesized evidence with care and re-review its individual research evidence to better judge the quality of the studies in the synthesis.

Publications That Report Scientific Evidence

When EBP team members begin looking for research evidence, they will find that this category of evidence can be broadly grouped into *summative research techniques* (meta-analysis and meta-synthesis) and *primary research designs* (experimental, quasi-experimental, non-experimental, and qualitative). Reviewers may also find secondary analyses that use data from primary studies. It is important that EBP teams recognize and appraise each evidence type and the relative strength it provides. The studies found under each broad design category provide nurses with a working knowledge of the properties, strengths, and limitations of research studies to enable nurses to judge the relative quality of evidence.

Summative Research Techniques

EBP teams generally consider themselves lucky when they uncover well-executed summative research techniques that apply to the practice question of interest. The two most prevalent techniques are meta-analysis and meta-synthesis. Table 6.1 outlines the defining features of these two techniques.

Table 6.1.   Defining Features of Summative Research Techniques

Summative Evidence	Description	Defining Features
Meta-analysis	Research technique that synthesizes and analyzes quantitative scientific evidence; narrower scope	■ uses statistical procedures to pool results from independent primary studies ■ usually includes experimental and/or quasi-experimental studies
Meta-synthesis	Research technique that synthesizes and analyzes qualitative scientific evidence; narrower scope	■ identification of key metaphors and concepts ■ interprets and translates findings ■ limited to qualitative studies

Meta-analysis

A *meta-analysis* is a type of scientific evidence that quantitatively synthesizes and analyzes the findings of multiple primary studies that have addressed a similar research question (Conn & Rantz, 2003). It involves applying statistics to pooled results from independent studies that are similar enough to combine. Meta-analyses present a summary of previous studies "using statistical techniques to transform findings of studies with related or identical hypotheses into a common metric and calculating the overall effect, the magnitude of effect, and sub-sample effects" (Whittemore, 2005, p. 57). A meta-analysis can be based on individual patient data from the primary studies, or each primary study can serve as a unit of analysis.

Combining a number of studies effectively creates one larger study to which statistical methods can be applied to more precisely determine the effect of interventions (Ciliska, Cullum, & Marks, 2001). A common metric, called an *effect size* (a measure of the strength of a relationship between two variables), is developed for each of the primary studies. A positive effect size indicates a positive relationship (as one variable increases, the second variable increases); a negative effect size indicates a negative relationship (as one variable increases or decreases, the second variable goes in the opposite direction).

An *overall summary statistic* combines and averages effect sizes across studies. An investigator should describe the method that determined the effect size and should help the reader interpret the statistic. Cohen's (1988) methodology for determining effect sizes includes the following strength of correlation ratings: trivial (ES = 0.01–0.09), low to moderate (0.10–0.29), moderate to substantial (0.30–0.49), substantial to very strong (0.50–0.69), very strong (0.70–0.89), and almost perfect (0.90–0.99)

An example of a meta-analysis is "A Meta-Analysis of Studies of Nurses' Job Satisfaction" (Zangaro & Soeken, 2007), which looked at the strength of the relationships between the job satisfaction of staff nurses and three constructs: autonomy, job stress, and nurse-physician collaboration.

Meta-synthesis

In contrast to quantitative research, qualitative research asks questions that draw on curiosity, involves a flexible repetitive process, aims at reflecting diversity rather than finding representative characteristics, and generates rather than collects data (Barbour & Barbour, 2003). Meta-synthesis, thought of as the qualitative counterpart to meta-analysis, employs a variety of methods to systematically review and integrate findings from qualitative studies (Sandelowski, 2006).

Meta-synthesis is similar to a multiple case study in which the primary qualitative studies form the individual cases (Jones, 2004). Meta-synthesis codes, charts, and maps the key metaphors and concepts in each qualitative study, and their relationships to each other are determined. This interpretive technique involves bringing together ideas that have been deconstructed in three meta-study processes: meta-data, meta-method, and meta-theory synthesis (Dixon-Woods, Agarwal, Jones, Young, & Sutton, 2005). The result is a complex synthesis that has the potential to broaden the ability to generalize findings of small sample qualitative studies so that they can apply to clinical situations (Whittemore, 2005).

The emphasis in qualitative research on individual experiences defies adding up those experiences, yet synthesis of findings from these studies is essential to enhancing the ability to generalize findings (Sandelowski, Docherty, & Emden, 1997). Hence, the aim of a meta-synthesis is not to produce a summary statistic, but rather to interpret and translate findings. For nurses who lack experience and expertise in critiquing qualitative studies, meta-syntheses aid not only assessing the rigor of individual studies but also the interpretation of findings.

An example of a qualitative meta-synthesis is "Parenting a child with chronic illness" (Coffey, 2006), which searched multiple online databases to yield 11 qualitative studies focusing on parenting a child with a chronic illness.

Primary Research

Most often, an EBP team retrieves reports of primary research studies. The team may also uncover secondary analyses of data gathered during the conduct of previous research studies. In secondary analysis, the researcher is able to test new hypotheses or ask new research questions using some of the data gathered in a prior study. Table 6.2 outlines the distinctive features of the various types of research evidence the team might uncover.

Table 6.2.   Distinctive Features of Research Studies

Design	Distinctive Features	Examples
Experimental	■ Randomization ■ Manipulation ■ Control	■ Randomized controlled trial
Quasi-experimental	■ No randomization ■ Some manipulation ■ Some control	■ Non-equivalent control group: posttest only or pretest-posttest ■ One group: posttest only or pretest-posttest ■ Untreated control, repeated measures ■ Repeated treatment where subjects serve as their own controls ■ Crossover design ■ Time series

Non-experimental	■ No randomization
	■ No manipulation
	■ Little control
		■ Descriptive
		   ▪ Exploratory
		   ▪ Survey
		   ▪ Descriptive comparative
		   ▪ Time dimensional
		■ Correlational

Qualitative	■ No randomization ■ No manipulation ■ Little control	■ Historical research ■ Grounded theory ■ Ethnographic ■ Phenomenological-hermeneutic

Experimental Studies

Experimental studies, or randomized controlled trials (RCTs), use the traditional scientific method. The investigator obtains verifiable, objective, research-based knowledge by observing or measuring in a manner such that resulting evidence is reproducible. Types of experimental designs that an EBP team might find during a literature search include pretest-posttest control group (the original or classic experimental design), posttest only comparison group, factorial, randomized block, nested, and crossover/repeated measures (Burns & Grove, 2005).

A true experimental study has three distinctive features: *randomization, control,* and *manipulation* (Polit & Beck, 2004). *Randomization* occurs when the researcher assigns subjects to a control or experimental group on a random basis, similar to the roll of dice. This ensures that each potential subject who meets inclusion criteria has the same probability of selection for the experiment. That is, people in the experimental and control groups will be, in a very broad sense, identical except for the introduction of the experimental intervention or treatment. This is important, because subjects who take part in an experiment serve as representatives of the population that the researcher feels the intervention or treatment may possibly benefit in the future.

Under optimal circumstances, the researcher and subjects are not aware of whether the subject has been randomized to the experimental group or the control group. This is *double-blinding.* For example, the subjects, their caregivers, or others involved in a study, would not be told whether the subject is receiving a vitamin supplement or a placebo (inactive substance). This is to minimize bias on the part of subjects and researchers. Sometimes, it may be possible to blind the subjects to the experimental treatment but not the investigator, who applies either the experimental treatment or a control treatment (e.g., comparing two patient educational strategies). This is *single-blinding.*

Manipulation is the researcher doing something to at least some of the subjects. An experimental treatment or intervention is applied to some subjects (the *experimental group*) and withheld from others (the *control group*) in an effort to influence some aspect of their health and well-being. The aspect that the researcher is trying to influence is the *dependent variable* (e.g., the experience of low back pain). The experimental treatment or intervention is the *independent variable*, or the action the researcher is going to take (e.g., application of low-level heat therapy) to try to change the dependent variable.

Control usually refers to the introduction of a control or comparison group, such as a group of subjects to which the experimental intervention or treatment is NOT applied. The goal is to compare the effect of the experimental intervention or treatment on the dependent variable in the control group against the effect of the same intervention or treatment on the dependent variable in the experimental group.

An example of an experimental study is "The Effect of Peer Counselors on Breastfeeding Rates in the Neonatal Intensive Care Unit: Results of a Randomized Controlled Trial" (Merewood, Chamberlain, Cook, Philipp, Malone, & Bauchner, 2006).

Quasi-experimental Studies

Quasi-experimental designs are similar to experimental designs in that they try to show that an intervention causes a particular outcome. Quasi-experimental studies are performed when it is not practical, ethical, or possible to randomly assign subjects to experimental and control groups. These studies involve some degree of investigator control as well as manipulation of an independent variable. However, they lack randomization, the key ingredient of experimental studies. Because randomization is absent, the researcher makes some effort to compensate for the lack of random assignment, such as using multiple groups or multiple waves of measurement (Trochim, 2006).

In cases where a particular intervention is effective, withholding that intervention would be unethical. In the same vein, it would not be practical to perform a study that requires more human, financial, and material resources than are available. There are times when neither patients nor geographical locations can be randomized. Consider the investigator who wants to study the effect of use of an alcohol-based hand disinfectant on vancomycin-resistant enterococcus acquisition rates. It would not be easy to randomize the use of disinfectant to individual patient rooms or to individual patients, because staff members would probably not agree to re-contaminate themselves before seeing a new patient (Harris, Bradham, Baumgarten, Zuckerman, Fink, & Perencevich, 2004).

Quasi-experimental designs that an EBP team might uncover during the course of its search include non-equivalent comparison group posttest only and non-equivalent comparison group pretest-posttest. The term *non-equivalent* means that not only is assignment non-random, but the researcher does not control assignment to groups. Hence, groups may be different and group differences may affect outcomes. Other quasi-experimental designs include one group posttest only, one group pretest-posttest, time-series, untreated control with repeated measures, repeated treatment where subjects serve as their own controls, crossover design (where the same subjects receive at different times both the experimental and the control intervention), and time series (Larson, 2005).

An example of a quasi-experimental study is "Effects of a Stroke Rehabilitation Education Programme for Nurses" (Booth, Hillier, Waters, & Davidson, 2005), which used a non-equivalent comparison group design to study the effects of a rehabilitation education program on the practice of nursing in two stroke rehabilitation units. An example of a quasi-experimental study using a design is "Effectiveness of Hand-Washing Teaching Programs for Families and Children in Paediatric Intensive Care Units" (Chen & Chiang, 2007).

Non-Experimental Studies

When reviewing evidence related to health-care questions, particularly inquiries of interest to nursing, EBP teams will find that most published studies are non-experimental in design. Non-experimental research involves the study of naturally occurring phenomena (groups, treatments, and individuals) without the introduction of an intervention. Subjects are not randomly assigned to different groups, there is no manipulation of variables, and the investigator is not always able to control aspects of the environment.

Two broad categories of non-experimental studies are *descriptive* and *correlational*. The basic question asked in descriptive research is: What are the quantifiable values of particular variables for a given set of subjects? The basic question asked in correlational research is: What is the relationship between two or more variables for a given set of subjects? One point to remember is that correlation *does not* infer causality.

Descriptive Designs

The intent of purely descriptive designs is, as the name implies, to *describe* characteristics of phenomena. There is no manipulation of variables and no attempt to determine that a particular intervention or characteristic causes a specific occurrence to happen. The investigators seek to provide the *who*, *what*, *where*, *when*, and *how* of particular persons, places, or things. An attempt is made to describe the answers to these questions in precisely measured terms. Statistical analysis is generally limited to frequencies and averages. Types of descriptive designs include exploratory, survey, descriptive comparative, and time-dimensional studies.

Exploratory and survey designs are quite common in nursing and health care. When little knowledge about the phenomenon of interest exists, these designs offer the greatest degree of flexibility. While new information is learned, the direction of the exploration may change. With exploratory designs, the investigator does not know enough about a phenomenon to identify variables of interest completely. Variables observed are as they happen; there is no researcher control. When investigators know enough about a particular phenomenon and can identify specific variables of interest, a descriptive survey design more fully describes the phenomenon. Questionnaire or interview techniques assess the variables of interest.

Descriptive comparative designs look at and describe differences in variables between or among two or more groups (Burns & Grove, 2005). Generally, descriptive statistics, such as frequency distributions and measures of central tendency (mean, median, and mode), are used to summarize these differences.

Time-dimensional designs look at "sequences and patterns of change, growth or trends over time" (Burns & Grove, 2005, p. 234). An EBP team should understand the concept of retrospective and prospective with respect to examining a phenomenon over time. In *retrospective* studies, the investigator looks at proposed causes and the effects that have already happened in order to learn from the past. In contrast, *prospective* studies examine causes that may have occurred in the past to anticipate effects that have not yet transpired. Time-dimensional designs that an EBP team may encounter include: *longitudinal*, a look at changes in the same subjects over time; *cross-sectional*, an examination of changes in groups of subjects over different stages of development; and *trends*, a study of changes in a population with respect to a particular phenomenon; (Burns & Grove, 2005).

When reviewing descriptive studies, an EBP team may encounter the following terms: case-control, cohort, and cross-sectional. *Case-control* studies involve comparing cases (subjects with a certain condition) with controls (subjects who lack that condition). *Cohort* studies look at a particular subset of a population from which different samples are taken at various points in time. *Cross-sectional* studies involve the collection of data at one particular point in time. Because unfamiliar terminology can divert the reviewer's attention from review of a study, an understanding of these terms should minimize confusion. An example of a descriptive design is "Sleep-Wake Disturbances and Quality of Life in Patients With Advanced Lung Cancer" (Vena et al., 2006).

Correlational Designs

Studies using correlational designs examine relationships among variables. The investigator gathers information on at least two variables, converts this information into numbers so that statistical analyses can be conducted, and runs a correlation between the two variables of interest using a statistical package to obtain a *correlation coefficient*—a number ranging from –1 to 1 (Sage, 2001). The correlation coefficient tells the *direction* of the association between the two variables. If the correlation coefficient is between 0 and 1, the correlation is positive, meaning that as one variable of interest increases, so does the second variable. A negative correlation is depicted by correlation coefficients between –1 and 0, meaning that as one variable increases, the other variable decreases. The correlation coefficient also tells the reader the strength or *magnitude* of the correlation. That is, the closer this coefficient is to 1 (if positive) or –1 (if negative), the stronger the association between the two variables.

Correlational designs include *descriptive correlational*, *predictive*, and *model testing* (Burns & Grove, 2005). Descriptive correlational designs seek to *describe* a relationship. Predictive correlational designs seek to *predict* relationships. Model testing designs seek to *test* the relationships put forth by a proposed causal model.

An example of a study that uses a predictive correlational design is "Perceived Readiness for Hospital Discharge in Adult Medical-Surgical Patients" (Weiss et al., 2007), which explored relationships among transition theory-related variables, such as the nature of the transition, patient characteristics, nursing therapeutics, and patterns of response to discharge.

Qualitative Designs

Qualitative designs represent a unique category of descriptive research in that they challenge the traditional scientific worldview. In effect, qualitative researchers design studies while conducting them, as opposed to conducting studies by design (Sandelowski & Barroso, 2003). Qualitative researchers summarize and interpret data to develop insights into the meaning of life experiences.

Examples of qualitative designs include historical research, grounded theory, ethnographic, phenomenological-hermeneutic, and case studies. *Historical* designs use narrative description or analysis of events that occurred in the remote or recent past to find answers to current questions (Burns & Grove, 2005). *Grounded theory* designs seek to examine social and psychological phases that characterize particular phenomena (Polit & Beck, 2004). *Ethnography* describes and analyzes characteristics of the ways of life of cultures or subcultures, and is of growing interest to nurses who seek to provide culturally competent care. *Hermeneutic phenomenology* is both a descriptive (phenomenological) methodology in that it lets a phenomenon speak for itself and an interpretive (hermeneutic) methodology in that it claims that all phenomena can be interpreted (van Manen, 2000). "Empathy, Inclusion, and Enclaves: The Culture of Care of People With HIV/AIDS and Nursing Implications" (Hodgson, 2006) is an example of a qualitative study that uses an ethnographic approach.

Because qualitative and quantitative research designs are complementary, many studies use a combination of both. Quantitative studies involve breaking the whole to examine each part and qualitative studies take a more holistic view and try to give meaning to the whole (Burns & Grove, 2005). Additionally, *triangulation* is the use of multiple research methodologies to study the same research question.

Interpreting Primary Research Evidence

To consider statistical information presented in reports of research evidence effectively, an EBP team needs a basic understanding of a study's *validity*, or soundness. Measures of validity include statistical conclusion validity, internal validity, external validity, and construct validity. The team should also understand how to interpret statistical measures of precision, that is, measures of central tendency, *p*-value, and confidence intervals.

Statistical Conclusion Validity

Statistical conclusion validity refers to legitimacy of conclusions about relationships and differences derived from statistical analysis of the data (Polit & Beck, 2004). Considerations addressed are statistical reliability, statistical significance, statistical power, and design precision (Garson, 2005; Polit & Beck). Although many staff nurses will not have the skill set to judge the proper use of statistics in the studies under review, they can look to see that the researchers have done so:

- Have the researchers established the statistical reliability of the measures used? Statistical reliability denotes the consistency of the measures obtained when a particular instrument is used and indicates the extent of random error in the measurement method.

- Have they discussed the possibility of *Type I* error—finding statistical significance when there is no true difference? Type I error arises when the researcher finds that differences between groups are significant when, in fact, differences are not significant. With Type I error, the null hypothesis (which states that there is no difference between the two groups) is rejected, when it should be accepted. Type I error is more likely to exist with a .05 level of significance than with a .01 level of significance. (Statistical significance is discussed later in this chapter as a measure of precision).

- Have the researchers considered the possibility of *Type II* error—failing to find statistical significance when there is a true difference? Type II error occurs when the null hypothesis is accepted as true (no significant differences between groups) when differences actually exist. Type II error is minimized when the statistical power of the study is high.

- Have the researchers considered *statistical power*—the ability to detect relationships and differences among variables, given that they actually exist? Adequate statistical power is dependent on sufficient sample size. Without a sufficient number of subjects, investigators would not be able to achieve adequate power to detect statistical significance. Although statistical power analysis is beyond the scope of this chapter, the EBP team should look for investigators to report the results of a power analysis to estimate their sample size.

- Do the researchers discuss the degree of *design precision* of the research project? Problems that can adversely affect design precision include: lack of standardization (inconsistency of conditions), insufficient training of research personnel, or inadequate monitoring procedures to ensure that the treatment is administered as planned (Polit & Beck, 2004).

Internal Validity

Internal validity is the degree to which observed changes in the dependent variable attribute to the experimental treatment or intervention, not other possible causes. Internal validity is particularly relevant to studies in which the researcher is trying to infer that the experimental intervention causes a particular effect or that a causal relationship exists (Trochim, 2006). An EBP team should question the degree to which there is evidence that there may be a competing explanation for observed results.

There are many threats to internal validity, all of which represent possible sources of bias. These include: *investigator bias,* such as the Hawthorne Effect, in which subjects alter their behavior because they are participating in a study, and not because of the research intervention; *attrition bias,* in which loss of subjects during a study affects the representative nature of the sample; and *selection bias,* which affects all nonrandom samples.

External Validity

External validity refers to the likelihood conclusions involving generalizations of research findings apply to other settings or samples. Simply, have the investigators concluded that their study would hold true for similar subjects in similar settings at other times (Trochim, 2006)? It is felt that "an increased focus on external validity of studies and generalizability of findings could increase the use of knowledge generated in those studies" (Ferguson, 2004, p. 16). An EBP team should question the degree to which study conclusions might reasonably hold true for its particular patient population and setting.

There are three major threats to external validity (Trochim, 2006). The researchers' generalization could be wrong in terms of person, place, or time. That is, they attempt to generalize findings from one group of persons to another, one clinical site to another setting, or one time to another in ways that may not be appropriate.

Construct Validity

Construct validity concerns the measurement of variables, specifically the legitimacy of assuming that what the investigators are measuring actually measures the construct of interest. A construct is a way of defining something. Construct validity refers to how well you translate your ideas into measures (Trochim, 2006). If the investigators define a measure in a way that is very different from how other researchers define the same measure, then the construct validity is suspect (Garson, 2005). Questions that a nurse might pose to get at threats to construct validity include: Did the researcher do a good job of defining the constructs? When the researchers say that they are measuring what they call *fatigue*, is that what they are really measuring?

Measures of Precision

Precision language describes populations and characteristics of populations. An EBP team should be very familiar with measures of central tendency (mean, median, and mode) and variation (standard deviation). The *mean* denotes the average value. Although a good measure of central tendency in normal symmetric distributions, the mean is misleading when there are skewed (asymmetric) distributions. The *median*, the number that lies at the midpoint of a distribution of values, is less sensitive to extreme scores and, therefore, of greater use in skewed distributions. The *mode* is the most frequently occurring value, and is the only measure of central tendency used with nominal (categorical) data. *Standard deviation*, a measure of variability that denotes the spread of the distribution, indicates the average variation of values from the mean.

Another measure of precision is statistical significance. To say that a result is statistically significant is to say that it is unlikely to have occurred by chance. The classic measure of statistical significance, the *p-value*, is a probability range from 0 to 1. It assumes that the *null hypothesis* (no difference between two variables) is true, and, if the *p*-value is below the significance level, then the null hypothesis is rejected. The smaller the *p*-value (the closer it is to 0), the more likely the result is statistically significant and the more likely one can reject the null hypothesis. In nursing literature, statistical significance is generally set at $p < .05$.

The concept of statistical significance is an important one, but should not be confused with the concept of clinical significance. Just because results are statistically significant does not mean that they have practical application to patient care. Statistically significant results are more likely to have clinical significance, but this is not always the case. In the same way, results that are not statistically significant (because of small sample sizes, for example) can still have clinical importance.

Although *p*-values are useful for investigators when planning how large a study needs to be to demonstrate a certain magnitude of effect, they fail to give clinicians the information they most need, that is, the range of values within which the true treatment effect is found (The Evidence-Based Teaching Tips Working Group, 2004). For this purpose, the confidence interval helps to specify precision.

What exactly is the *confidence interval* (CI)? This measure of precision is an estimate of a range of values within which the actual value lies. The CI contains an upper and lower limit. A 95% CI is the range of values within which a nurse can be 95% confident that the actual values in a given population fall between the lower and upper limits (Klardie, Johnson, McNaughton, & Meyers, 2004).

Appraising the Strength and Quality of Research Evidence

The use of rating scales assists the critical appraisal of evidence. Rating scales present a structured way to differentiate evidence of varying strengths and quality. The underlying assumption is that recommendations from strong evidence of high quality would be more likely to represent best practices than evidence of lower strength and less quality. Tables 6.3 and 6.4 present the rating schemes used in the JHNEBP process to evaluate the strength and quality of *research* evidence.

Table 6.3.   Strength of Research Evidence Rating Scheme

LEVEL	TYPE OF EVIDENCE
I	Evidence obtained from an experimental study/randomized controlled trial (RCT) or meta-analysis of RCTs
II	Evidence obtained from a quasi-experimental study
III	Evidence obtained from a non-experimental study, qualitative study, or meta-synthesis

Table 6.4.   Quality Rating Scheme for Research Evidence

Grade	Research Evidence
A: High	Consistent results with sufficient sample, adequate control, and definitive conclusions; consistent recommendations based on extensive literature review that includes thoughtful reference to scientific evidence
B: Good	Reasonably consistent results; sufficient sample, some control, with fairly definitive conclusions; reasonably consistent recommendations based on fairly comprehensive literature review that includes some reference to scientific evidence
C: Low/Major flaw	Little evidence with inconsistent results; insufficient sample size; conclusions cannot be drawn.

Grading Quality of Research Evidence

The large number of checklists and rating instruments available for grading the quality of research studies presents a challenge to an EBP team. Tools to appraise the quality of scientific evidence usually contain explicit criteria, with varying degrees of specificity according to the evidence type. Nurses often do not have the comprehensive knowledge of methodological strengths and limitations required to interpret these criteria. It is important for an EBP team to involve someone with knowledge of interpretation of research and statistics, often a nurse with a doctoral degree.

Because the development of any EBP skill set is evolutionary, the JHNEBP Model uses a broadly defined quality rating scale. This provides structure for a nurse reviewer, yet allows for the application of critical-thinking skills specific to the team's knowledge and experience reviewing the evidence being critiqued. The application of this scale, shown in Table 6.4, accommodates qualitative judgments related to both research and non-research evidence.

Judgments of quality should be relative. That is, the quality grade given for each piece of evidence reviewed is by comparison with the body of evidence reviewed by each member, past and present—independently and as a group member. As the group gains experience reading and appraising research, the members' comfort level in making this determination will likely improve.

Rating Strength of Research Evidence

Research evidence, when well-executed (of good to high quality), is generally given a higher strength rating than other evidence. When appraising individual research studies, three major components come into play: *study design*, which is usually classified as experimental, quasi-experimental, non-experimental, and qualitative; *study quality*, which refers to study methods and execution; and *directness*, or the extent to which subjects, interventions, and outcome measures are similar to those of interest (GRADE Working Group, 2004).

When appraising overall evidence reviewed, a fourth component is added: *consistency*, or similarities in the size and/or direction of estimated effects across studies (GRADE Working Group, 2004). Identification of study designs and examination of *threats* to validity specific to the evidence type will help an EBP team to determine the overall strength and quality of research evidence.

Meta-analyses

The strength of the evidence on which recommendations are made within a meta-analytic design depends on the type and quality of studies included in the meta-analysis as well as their management within the meta-analysis process (Conn & Rantz, 2003). The strongest meta-analyses contain only randomized controlled trials. Evidence from these studies is Level I evidence. Some meta-analyses include data from quasi-experimental or non-experimental studies; hence, evidence would be only Level II or III in strength. The quality, clarity, and completeness of information presented in primary studies strongly affect the conduct of a meta-analysis (Burns & Grove, 2005). For an EBP team to evaluate evidence obtained from a meta-analysis, the report of the meta-analysis must be detailed enough for the reader to understand the studies included.

Meta-analyses reports should clearly identify how decisions were made to include or exclude studies. Investigators should also give a clear description of sound literature search strategies that include both computerized database explorations and hand searches of journals and reference lists of retrieved studies (Acton, 2001). EBP teams should use caution when reviewing meta-analyses that include findings published only in peer-reviewed journals, because these are likely to overestimate the effect size (Conn, 2004; Cowan, 2004). This overestimation results because studies without statistically significant findings are published less often than those with statistically significant findings. Some meta-analyses, to be more comprehensive, extend their review to unpublished data and unpublished studies reported in abstracts and dissertations.

To interpret evidence from meta-analyses, the team needs a basic understanding of how to interpret the summary statistic, or mean effect size. An *effect size* is the statistical relationship between two variables under consideration, or the size of the between-group differences with respect to some characteristic of interest (Polit & Beck, 2004). The *summary statistic* provides information about the existence of relationships between variables and, if links exist, the magnitude of such relationships. To aid in interpretation, the effect size is often expressed in terms of direction (positive, negative, or zero) and magnitude (high, medium, or small).

Experimental Studies

The strength of evidence is the highest, or Level I, when derived from a well-designed RCT on the question of interest or from a meta-analysis of RCTs that supports the same finding in different samples of the same population (See Table 6.2). An EBP team usually acquires these findings from the critical review of well-executed summative research summaries that draw their recommendations from well-designed RCTs.

Internal validity refers to the extent to which inferences regarding cause and effect are true. Internal validity is only relevant to studies that try to establish causal relationships. Potential threats to internal validity specific to experimental studies can be found in history, maturation, testing, and instrumentation (Polit & Beck, 2004). Questions a nurse may pose to uncover potential threats to internal validity include: Did some historical event occur during the course of the study that may have influenced the results of the study? Are there processes occurring within subjects over the course of the study because of the passage of time (maturation) rather than a result of the experimental intervention? Could the pretest have influenced the subject's performance on the posttest? Were the measurement instruments and procedures the same for both points of data collection?

External validity refers to the extent that results will hold true across different subjects, settings, and procedures. Potential threats to external validity in experimental studies relate to setting selection, patient selection, and characteristics of randomized patients; the difference between the trial protocol and routine practices, outcome measures and follow-up; and adverse effects of the treatment (Rothwell, 2005). Questions a nurse may pose to uncover potential threats to external validity include: How confident am I that the study findings can transfer from the sample to the entire population? Did subjects have inherent differences even before manipulation of the independent variable (selection bias)? Are participants responding in a certain way because they know they are being observed (the Hawthorne effect)? Are there researcher behaviors or characteristics that may influence the subject's responses (experimenter effect)? In multi-institutional studies, were there variations in how study coordinators at various sites managed the trial? Did following subjects more frequently or having them take diagnostic tests affect the outcomes in unpre-dicted ways? Did the study have a high dropout rate, affecting the representative nature of the sample? Is the sample size adequate?

Overall validity of an experimental study depends on the extent to which con-trol; avoidance of systematic error; and minimization of random, or chance, error is achieved (Blair, 2004). Problems can result when there is an imbalanced distribution of unknown or unrecognized causes of the outcome of the experimental treatment or intervention. For example, some initial characteristics of the sample (age, birth weight, and race) may have unrecognized disparities that have a clinically signifi-cant effect on the outcome. This is especially true in heterogeneous (dissimilar) or very small samples.

Quasi-experimental Studies

The strength of evidence gained from well-designed quasi-experimental studies is less than that of experimental studies. However, quasi-experimental studies are best when ethical considerations, practical issues, and feasibility prohibit the con-duct of RCTs. For that reason, the strength of evidence recommendation rating for a well-designed quasi-experimental study is Level II (See Table 6.3).

As with experimental studies, threats to internal validity characteristic of quasi-experimental studies include maturation, testing, and instrumentation, with the additional threats of history and selection (Polit & Beck, 2004). The occurrence of external events at the same time (threat of history) can affect subject response to the investigational intervention or treatment. Additionally, when groups are not as-signed randomly, the very nature of nonequivalent groups is such that there may be preexisting differences that affect the outcome.

In terms of external validity, threats associated with sampling design, such as patient selection and characteristics of non-randomized patients, affect the general findings. External validity improves if the researcher uses random selection of sub-jects, even if random assignment to groups is not possible.

Non-Experimental and Qualitative Studies

The strength of evidence gained from well-designed non-experimental studies and qualitative studies is the lowest rung of the research evidence ladder (Level III), but is still higher than that of non-research evidence. Questions of internal validity do not apply when reviewing descriptive designs (quantitative or qualitative).

When looking for potential threats to external validity, a nurse can pose the questions described under experimental studies. In addition, the nurse may ask additional questions, such as: Did the researcher attempt to control for extraneous variables with the use of careful subject selection criteria? Did the researcher attempt to minimize the potential for socially acceptable responses by the subject? Did the study rely on documentation as the source of data? In methodological studies (developing, testing, and evaluating research instruments and methods), were the test subjects selected from the population for which the test will be used? Was the survey response rate high enough to generalize findings to the target population? For historical research studies, are the data authentic and genuine?

Qualitative studies offer one additional challenge—it is often difficult for the reader to locate findings. Problems that lead to difficulties identifying qualitative research findings include misrepresentation of data as findings, misrepresentation of analysis as findings, misuse of quotes and incidents, problems ascertaining what the researchers mean when they state that something is a pattern or a theme, conceptual confusion or drifting from one concept to another when presenting findings (Sandelowski & Barroso, 2002).

Meta-syntheses (Level III Evidence)

Evaluating and synthesizing qualitative research presents a variety of challenges. Even seasoned researchers find qualitative meta-synthesis to be a complex exercise in interpretation (Sandelowski, Docherty, & Emden, 1997). It is, therefore, not surprising that clinical nurses often feel at a loss when it comes to assessing the quality of meta-synthesis. Approaching these reviews from a broad perspective allows a nurse to look for indicators of quality that both quantitative and qualitative summative research techniques have in common.

Explicit search strategies, inclusion and exclusion criteria, methodological details (not only of the included studies, but also of the conduct of the meta-synthesis itself), and how the reviewer manages study quality should all be noted. Similar to other summative modalities, a "meta-synthesis should be undertaken by a team of experts, since the application of multiple perspectives to the processes of study appraisal, coding, charting, mapping, and interpretation may result in additional insights, and thus in a more complete interpretation of the subject of the review" (Jones, 2004, p. 277).

Nurses need to keep in mind that judgments related to study strengths and weaknesses as well as the suitability of recommendations for the target population are both context-specific and dependent on the question asked. There will be conditions or circumstances, such as clinical setting or time of day, that are relevant to determining the applicability of a particular recommended intervention.

An example of a systematic review that includes a qualitative meta-synthesis is "Role Development and Effective Practice in Specialist and Advanced Practice Roles in Acute Hospital Settings: Systematic Review and Meta-Synthesis" (Jones, 2005), which reported on 14 studies that examined barriers and facilitators to role development and/or effective practice in specialist and advanced nursing roles.

Tips for Reading Research

Nurses engaging in EBP activities should be educated readers and interpreters of research publications. The completeness of a research report and the reader's ability to understand the meaning of terms used in the report can help or hinder an EBP team's efforts. Standards exist for the writing of research articles; however, the degree to which journals demand adherence to these standards varies. Essential elements of published research include the title, abstract, introduction, method, results, discussion, and conclusion (Lunsford & Lunsford, 1996). Readers will find that research reports do not always clearly delineate these sections with headers, although the elements may be present. For example, there is not typically a heading for the introduction or conclusion of a research report.

The Title

The title presents a starting point in determining whether the article has potential to be included in an EBP review. Ideally, the title should be informative and should help the reader to understand what type of study is being reported. A well-chosen title states what was done, to whom it was done, and how it was done. Consider the previously mentioned title "The Effect of Peer Counselors on Breastfeeding Rates in the Neonatal Intensive Care Unit: Results of a Randomized Controlled Trial" (Merewood, Chamberlain, Cook, Philipp, Malone, & Bauchner, 2006). The reader is immediately apprised of what was done (a peer counselor intervention), to whom it was done (breastfed neonates in the neonatal intensive care unit), and how it was done (a randomized controlled trial).

Often articles germane to an EBP question are skipped because the title does not give a clue as to its relevance. For example, consider the title "A Magnet Community Hospital: Fewer Barriers to Nursing Research Utilization" (Karkos & Peters, 2006). Although the reader will have an idea that the article concerns research utilization by nurses (*what* and *by whom*) in a Magnet community hospital (*where*), the title does not give any indication that this is a report of a research study using a descriptive survey design. The title is more reflective of an opinion piece than of a research report.

The Abstract

The abstract is usually located after the title and author section and is graphically set apart by use of a box, shading, or italics. A good abstract contains information about a study's purpose, method, results, conclusions, and clinical relevance. Huck (2004, p. 14) writes that "an abstract gives you a thumbnail sketch of a study, thus allowing you to decide whether the article fits into your area of interest," but cautions that there are dangers in thinking that one can read only the abstract and forego reading the entire article. The abstract should serve as a screening device only.

If the abstract appears to be relevant, then an examination of the introduction should occur. The introduction contains the background as well as a problem statement that tells why the investigators have chosen to conduct the particular study. Background is best presented within the context of a current literature review, and the author should identify the knowledge gap between what is known and what the study seeks. A clear, direct statement of purpose should be included as well as a statement of expected results or hypotheses. The statement of purpose is often, although not always, located immediately before the article's first main heading.

The Conclusion

The conclusion should contain a brief restatement of the experimental results and implications of study (Lunsford & Lunsford, 1996). If there is not a separate header for the conclusion, it usually falls at the end of the discussion section.

The Method

This section describes how a study is conducted (study procedures) in sufficient detail so that a reader could replicate the study, if desired. For example, if the intervention was administration of a placebo, the nature of the placebo should be stated. An investigator should identify the intended study population and provide a description of inclusion and exclusion criteria. How subjects were recruited and demographic characteristics of those who actually took part in the study should be included. In addition, if instrumentation was used, the method section should present evidence of instrument quality, even if well-known published tools are used. Finally, the report should contain a description of how data were collected and analyzed.

The Results

Study results list the findings of the data analysis and should not contain commentary. Give particular attention to figures and tables, which are the heart of most papers. Look to see whether results report statistical versus clinical significance and look up unfamiliar terminology, symbols, or logic.

The Discussion

Results should be tied to material in the introduction. The research questions should be answered, and meaning should be given to the results. The main weaknesses, or limitations, of the study should be identified and the broad implications of the findings should be stated.

The reviewer should be cautioned that writers might use language to sway the reader. Researchers can overstate their findings or use an assertive sentence in a way that makes it sound like a well-established fact (Graham, 1957). Carefully view vague expressions similar to "It is generally believed that ..."

The Overall Report

The parts of the research article should be highly interconnected and provide sufficient information so that the reviewer can make an informed judgment about the connections. Any hypotheses should flow directly from the review of literature. Results should support arguments presented in the discussion and conclusion sections.

An EBP team should be aware of duplicate publication, that is, more than one publication that reports findings from the same research study. "Duplicate publication of original research is particularly problematic, since it can result in inadvertent double counting or inappropriate weighting of the results of a single study, which distorts the available evidence" (International Committee of Medical Journal Editors, 2006, IIID2).

A Practical Tool for Appraising Research Evidence

The JHNEBP Research Evidence Appraisal (Appendix F) gauges the strength and quality of recommendations made by research evidence. The front of the tool contains questions to guide the team in determining the level of strength of recommendations and the quality of the primary studies included in the review. Strength of recommendations is higher (Level I) with evidence from at least one well-designed randomized controlled trial (RCT) than from at least one well-designed quasi-experimental (Level II,) non-experimental (Level III), or qualitative (Level III) study. The reverse side of the tool contains descriptors of the research types as well as the scale used to determine quality of the research.

An EBP team can use the JHNEBP Individual Evidence Summary (Appendix H) to summarize key findings from each of the individual pieces of evidence appraised. This allows the team to view pertinent information related to each source (author, evidence type, sample type and size, results and recommendations, limitations, and strength and quality ratings) in one document.

An EBP team can use the JHNEBP Overall Evidence Summary (Appendix I) to document the quantity, strength, and quality of all the evidence reviewed and to develop recommendations for changes in processes or systems of care.

Recommendations for Nurse Leaders

Knowledge gained from research studies is valuable only to the extent that it is shared with others and appropriately translated into practice. Professional standards have long held that nurses need to integrate the best available evidence, including research findings, into guiding practice decisions. Research articles can be intimidating to novice and expert nurses alike. Reading scientific papers is "partly a matter of experience and skill, and partly learning the specific vocabulary of a field" (McNeal, 2005, ¶1). Nurse leaders can best support EBP by providing clinicians with the knowledge and skills necessary to appraise research evidence. Only through continual learning can clinicians gain the confidence needed to incorporate the evidence gleaned from research into the day-to-day care of individual patients.

References

Acton, G. L. (2001). Meta-analysis: A tool for evidence-based practice. *AACN Clinical Issues Advanced Practice in Acute Critical Care, 12*(4), 539-545.

Barbour, R. S., & Barbour, M. (2003). Evaluating and synthesizing qualitative research: The need to develop a distinctive approach. *Journal of Evaluation in Clinical Practice, 9*(2), 179-186.

Blair, E. (2004). Gold is not always good enough: The shortcomings of randomization when evaluating interventions in small heterogeneous samples. *Journal of Clinical Epidemiology, 57,* 1219-1222.

Booth, J., Hillier, V. F., Waters, K. R., & Davidson, I. (2005). Effects of a stroke rehabilitation education programme for nurses. *Journal of Advanced Nursing, 49*(5), 365-473.

Burns, N., & Grove, S. K. (2005). *The practice of nursing research* (5th ed). St. Louis, MO: Elsevier Saunders.

Chen, Y. C., & Chiang, L. C. (2007). Effectiveness of hand-washing teaching programs for families of children in paediatric intensive care units. *Journal of Clinical Nursing, 16*(6), 1173-1179.

Ciliska, D., Cullum, N., & Marks, S. (2001). Evaluation of systematic reviews of treatment or prevention interventions. *Evidence-Based Nursing, 4,* 100-104.

Coffey, J. S. (2006). Parenting a child with chronic illness: A metasynthesis. *Pediatric Nursing, 32,* 51-59.

Cohen, J. (1988). *Statistical power analysis for the behavioral sciences.* New York: Academic Press.

Conn, V. S. (2004). Meta-analysis research. *Journal of Vascular Nursing, 22,* 51-52.

Conn, V., & Rantz, M. (2003). Research methods: Managing primary study quality in meta-analyses. *Research in Nursing and Health, 26,* 322-333.

Cowan, P.A. (2004). Advancing evidence-based practice through meta-analysis. *Nephrology Nursing Journal, 31*(3), 343-344, 347.

Dixon-Woods, M., Agarwal, S., Jones, D., Young, B., & Sutton, A. (2005). Synthesizing qualitative and quantitative evidence: A review of possible methods. *Journal of Health Services Research & Policy, 10*(1), 45-53.

The Evidence-Based Medicine Teaching Tips Working Group; Montori, V. M., Kleinbart, J., Newman, T. B., Keitz, S., Wyer, P. C., Moyer, V., & Guyatt, G. (2004). Tips for learners of evidence-based medicine: 2. Measures of precision (confidence intervals). *Canadian Medical Association Journal, 171*(6), 611-615.

Ferguson, L. (2004). External validity, generalizability, and knowledge utilization. *Journal of Nursing Scholarship, 36*(1), 16-22.

Garson, G. D. (2005). *PA 765. Statnotes. An on-line textbook.* Retrieved August 20, 2006, from http://www2.chass.ncsu.edu/garson/pa765/statnote.htm

GRADE Working Group. (2004). Systems for grading the quality of evidence and the strength of recommendations I: Critical appraisal of existing approaches. *BMC Health Services Research, 4*(1), 38.

Graham, C. D. (1957). *A dictionary of useful research phrases.* Retrieved August 23, 2006, from http://www.flyzhy.org/research/dictionary_research.html

Harris, A. D., Bradham, D. D., Baumgarten, M., Zuckerman, I. H., Fink, J. C., & Perencevich. E. N. (2004). The use and interpretation of quasi-experimental studies in infectious diseases. *Clinical Infectious Diseases, 38,* 1586-1591.

Hodgson, I. (2006) Empathy, inclusion and enclaves: The culture of care of people with HIV/AIDS and nursing implications. *Journal of Advanced Nursing, 55,* 283-290.

Huck, S. W. (2004). *Reading statistics and research* (4th ed.). Boston: Pearson Allyn and Bacon.

International Committee of Medical Journal Editors. (2006). *Uniform requirements for manuscripts submitted to biomedical journals: Writing and editing for biomedical publication.* Retrieved August 20, 2006, from http://www.ICMJE.org

Jones, M. L. (2004). Application of systematic review methods to qualitative research: practical issues. *Journal of Advanced Nursing, 48*(3), 271-278.

Jones, M. L. (2005). Role development and effective practice in specialist and advanced practice roles in acute hospital settings: Systematic review and meta-synthesis. *Journal of Advanced Nursing, 49*(2), 191-209.

Karkos, B., & Peters, K. (2006). A Magnet community hospital. Fewer barriers to nursing research utilization. *Journal of Nursing Administration, 36(7/8),* 377-382.

Klardie, K. A., Johnson, J., McNaughton, M. A., & Meyers, W. (2004). Integrating the principles of evidence-based practice into clinical practice. *Journal of the American Academy of Nurse Practitioners, 16*(3), 98-105.

Larson, E. (2005). *Research designs. Course notes M6728, theory and research in applied sciences and nursing.* Retrieved on August 20, 2006, from www.columbia.edu/~ell23/outline6.html

Lunsford, T. R., & Lunsford, B. R. (1996). Research forum. How to critically read a journal research article. *Journal of Prosthetics and Orthotics, 8,* 24-31.

McNeal, A. (2005). *How to read a scientific research paper—a four-step guide for students and for faculty.* Retrieved August 20, 2006, from http://helios.hampshire.edu/~apmNS/design/RESOURCES/HOW_READ.html

Merewood, A., Chamberlain, L. B., Cook, J. T., Philipp, B. L., Malone, K., & Bauchner, H. (2006). The effect of peer counselors on breastfeeding rates in the neonatal intensive care unit: Results of a randomized controlled trial. *Archives in Pediatric Adolescent Medicine, 160,* 681-685

Polit, D. F., & Beck, C. T. (2004). *Nursing research. Principles and methods* (7th ed.). Philadelphia: Lippincott Williams & Wilkens.

Rothwell, P. M. (2005). External validity of randomized controlled trials: "To whom do the results of this trial apply?" *Lancet, 365,* 82-93.

Sage, N. A. (2001). Elements of a research study. Accessed August 20, 2006, from http://www.psy.pdx.edu/PsyTutor/Tutorials/Research/Elements/

Sandelowski, M. (2006). "Meta-jeopardy:" The crisis of representation in qualitative metasynthesis. *Nursing Outlook, 54*(1), 10-6.

Sandelowski, M., & Barroso, J. (2002). Finding the findings in qualitative studies. *Journal of Nursing Scholarship, 34,* 213-219.

Sandelowski, M., & Barroso, J. (2003). Writing the proposal for a qualitative research methodology project. *Qualitative Health Research, 13,* 781-820.

Sandelowski, M., Docherty, S., & Emden, C. (1997). Qualitative metasynthesis: Issues and techniques. *Research in Nursing & Health, 20,* 365-371.

Trochim, W. M. K. (2006). *The research methods knowledge base* (2nd ed.). Retrieved August 20, 2006, from http://www.socialresearchmethods.net/kb/

van Manen, M. (2000). *Glossary of terms in phenomenology.* Retrieved on August 20, 2006, from http://www.phenomenologyonline.com/glossary/glossary.html

Vena, C., Parker, K. P., Allen, R., Bliwise, D. L., Jain, S., & Kimble, L. (2006). Sleep-wake disturbances and quality of life in patients with advanced lung cancer. *Oncology Nursing Forum, 33,* 761-769.

Weiss, M. E., Piacentine, L. B., Lokken, L., Ancona, J., Archer, J., Gresser, S., et al. (2007). Perceived readiness for hospital discharge in adult medical-surgical patients. *Clinical Nurse Specialist, 21*(1), 31-34.

Whittemore, R. (2005). Combining evidence in nursing research: Methods and implications. *Nursing Research, 54*(1), 56-62.

Zangaro, G. A., & Soeken, K. L., (2007). A meta-analysis of studies of nurses' job satisfaction; *Research in Nursing & Health, 30,* 445-458.

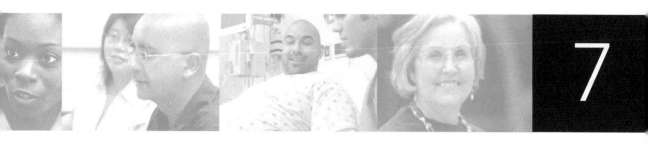

7

Evidence Appraisal:
Non-Research

Despite the inclusion of research in baccalaureate and master's nursing education, the comfort level with reading and applying research studies varies among new graduates and experienced nurses. Moreover, when research evidence does not exist, or is insufficient to answer the practice question, many nurses do not have experience with appraising other non-research evidence that has the potential to inform their practice.

Non-research evidence encompasses a broad range of categories. Such evidence includes Carper's (1978) personal, aesthetic, and ethical knowledge domains, which are reflected through the expertise, experience, and values of individual practitioners as well as the lived experiences and values of patients and their families. Opinions of recognized experts in the field (individual and collective professional authorities or consensus groups), as well as discoveries made through human and organizational (both individual and collective) experiences, add depth and breadth to the evidence review. For the purposes of this chapter, non-research evidence is divided into summative reviews of research evidence, expert opinion, human and organizational experience, practitioner experience and expertise, and patient experience. This chapter's objectives are to identify the types of non-research evidence and to describe strategies for evaluating non-research evidence.

The chapter closes with recommendations to clinical nurse leaders for building nurses' capacity to examine their practice with a thoughtful review and consideration of non-research evidence.

Summaries of Research Evidence

Summarized research evidence, such as integrative reviews or literature reviews, are an excellent source of support relevant to the practice question. These publications review and synthesize all research (not just experimental studies), although they themselves are not research evidence. Rather, they are non-research evidence because they reflect appraisal of the evidence and interpretation of the included studies. This summarized evidence is distinctly different from a meta-analysis or systematic review conducted by a team of experts (see Chapter 6).

Although many reports claim to summarize a particular phenomenon of interest, this chapter discusses two formalized methods of research review: systematic reviews and clinical practice guidelines. While systematic reviews usually limit their scope to scientific evidence, clinical practice guidelines often include non-research evidence to support recommendations. These publications can be very helpful for nurses on an EBP team who may have limited time and/or expertise to review large numbers of research studies. Table 7.1 presents defining features of various summative research reviews:

Table 7.1.   Defining Features of Summative Research Reviews

Summative Evidence	Description	Defining Features
Systematic Review	Review of research evidence related to a specific clinical question	Employs comprehensive search strategies, and rigorous appraisal methods can cover a range of research studies

Summative Evidence	Description	Defining Features
Clinical Practice Guidelines	Review of research and non-research evidence	Systematically developed statements to guide patient care decisions for specific clinical circumstances
		Combines research findings, provider expertise, and patient preferences

Published reports of quantitative research integrations are numerous. Notable efforts include *The Cochrane Collaboration*, an international non-profit organization that produces and disseminates systematic reviews of health-care interventions, and *Worldviews on Evidence-Based Nursing*, a peer-reviewed journal developed by The Honor Society of Nursing, Sigma Theta Tau International. A less prominent, but growing, effort to integrate and synthesize findings from qualitative research (Popay, 2006) exists; however, qualitative terms, such as meta-synthesis, grounded theory, and phenomenology, continue to be absent from the Cochrane glossary (Green & Higgins, 2005).

Systematic Reviews

Systematic reviews summarize critically appraised research evidence (usually experimental and quasi-experimental trials) related to a specific question. These reviews employ only comprehensive search strategies and rigorous transparent appraisal methods. Use of specific systematic methods in the review process helps minimize bias. A single expert or group of individuals experienced in the particular topic under review often performs these summaries.

Systematic reviews differ from the more traditional, but unsystematic, narrative literature reviews. Narrative literature reviews often contain references to research studies, but they do not critically appraise, evaluate, and summarize the relative merits of the studies under review. True systematic reviews address both the strengths and the limitations of each study included in the review.

Systematic review is interchangeable with *evidence report*. The Agency for Healthcare Research and Quality (AHRQ, formerly the Agency for Health Care

Policy and Research) awards 5-year contracts to institutions in the United States and Canada to serve as Evidence-based Practice Centers (EPCs). EPCs review scientific literature on clinical, behavioral, organizational, and financing topics to produce evidence reports and technology assessments (AHRQ, 2007). Additionally, EPCs conduct research on systematic review methodology.

To draw conclusions about the evidence collected, systematic reviews use explicit, well-defined, and reproducible strategies to identify, retrieve, and appraise research for relevance and validity (quality), for data extraction and synthesis, and for interpretation (Ciliska, Cullum, & Marks, 2001). These reviews may include the statistical methods of meta-analysis if primary studies meet certain assumptions (Whittemore, 2005).

A reader should not differentiate between a systematic review and a narrative literature review based on the title of the article. Often the title will state that the article presents a literature review when it is a systematic literature review. An example is "Failure to Rescue: A Literature Review" (Schmid, Hoffman, Happ, Wolf, & DeVita, 2007), which presents clear descriptions of methods of literature retrieval as well as synthesis and appraisal of studies included in the review.

Sometimes systematic reviews are *integrative reviews*, which include the systematic analysis and synthesis of research on a targeted topic. Not limited to randomized controlled trials, the integrative review can cover a range of experimental, quasi-experimental, and non-experimental studies. An example is "Integrative Review of Parenting in Nursing Research" (Gage, Everett, & Bullock, 2006), which synthesized and analyzed 17 published, peer-reviewed nursing research studies on parenting.

Clinical Practice Guidelines

Clinical practice guidelines (CPGs) represent another form of systematically developed statements that help inform patient care decision making in particular clinical situations (Institute of Medicine, 1992). Groups of experts who combine evidence from three sources (research findings, clinician expertise, and patient preferences) to develop best practice recommendations write CPGs (Hines et al., 2003). CPGs provide a body of evidence synthesized by interdisciplinary teams of experts for practitioners to manage patient care issues in the context of patient preferences and clinical expertise (Kent & Fineout-Overholt, 2007).

To help practitioners determine the quality of CPGs, the Institute of Medicine identified eight desirable attributes, which include validity, reliability and reproducibility, clinical applicability, clinical flexibility, clarity, documentation, development by a multidisciplinary process, and plans for review (Institute of Medicine, 1992). Many of these attributes were absent from published guidelines, resulting in the Conference on Guideline Standardization to promote guideline quality and to facilitate guideline implementation (Shiffman et al., 2003). The Appraisal of Guidelines Research and Evaluation (AGREE) Collaboration, using a guideline appraisal instrument with documented reliability and validity, found that the availability of background information was the strongest predictor of guideline quality, and that high-quality guidelines were more often produced by government-supported organizations or a structured, coordinated program (Fervers et al., 2005).

The National Guideline Clearinghouse (NGC), an initiative of the Agency for Healthcare Research and Quality (AHRQ), U.S. Department of Health and Human Services, has developed criteria designed to ensure rigor in developing and maintaining published guidelines (NGC, 2005). Included in these criteria are requirements that the clinical practice guideline

- include systematically developed statements that contain recommendations, strategies, or information that assists health-care practitioners and patients in making decisions

- be officially sponsored by one or more medical specialty associations, relevant professional societies, public or private organizations, government agencies, or health-care organizations or plans

- has a corroborative, verifiable documentation of a systematic literature search and review of existing research evidence published in peer reviewed journals

- has been developed, reviewed, or revised within the last 5 years and is available in print or electronic form in the English language

These rigorous standards are one of the reasons why the NGC is an excellent source of high quality guidelines. An example of a set of guidelines that meets the exacting requirements of the NGC is "Evidence-Based Guidelines for Cardiovascular Disease Prevention in Women" (Mosca et al., 2004).

Interpreting Evidence From Summative Reviews

When reading summative research reviews, an EBP team should look for desirable attributes that would indicate that the research review meets acceptable standards. Although a variety of desirable characteristics exists for each of the major research review methods, there are shared features that a nurse can identify when reading any summative research review. Table 7.2 lists the features that provide a framework for an EBP team to make decisions regarding the merits of recommendations made in a summative review:

Table 7.2. Desirable Attributes of Summative Documents Used to Answer an EBP Question

Attribute	Description
Applicability to phenomenon of interest	Does the summative document address the particular practice question of interest (same population, same setting)?
Comprehensiveness of search strategy	Do the authors identify search strategies that move beyond the typical databases, such as MEDLINE and CINAHL? Are published and unpublished works included?
Clarity of method	Do the authors clearly specify how decisions were made to include and exclude studies from the analysis, and how data were analyzed?
Unity and consistency of findings	Is there cohesive organization of study findings such that meaningful separation and synthesis of relevant concepts are clear to the reader? Does the publication contain logically organized tables with consistent information relative to the applicability of findings?

Attribute	Description
Management of study quality	Do the authors clearly describe how the review manages study quality?
Transparency of limitations	Are methodological limitations disclosed?
Believability of conclusions	Do the conclusions appear to be based on the evidence and capture the complexity of the clinical phenomenon?
Collective expertise	Was the review and synthesis done by a single individual with expertise or a group of experts?

*Adapted from Whittemore (2005), Conn (2004), and Stetler et al., (1998).

Similar to reports of primary studies, summative research reports should be carefully read, with readers making independent assessments of whether findings have been appropriately interpreted in the discussion portion of the report (Conn, 2004). Each team member should discuss his or her assessment with the group to reach a consensus regarding the appropriateness of the interpretation. When something of particular interest is found, the team should review the primary research report according to the methods discussed in Chapter 6.

Systematic Reviews (Level I, II, III, or IV Evidence)

The Cochrane Collaboration publishes the Cochrane Database of Systematic Reviews, which has rapidly grown over time. The Cochrane Reviewer's Handbook (2006) is considered "the most highly developed methodological source of systematic reviews" (Stevens, 2002, p. 232). This guide helps review writers be both systematic and explicit in developing their clinical question and in finding its answers (Alderson, Green, & Higgins, 2005). Although the work of the Cochrane Collaboration began with randomized controlled trials, it has expanded to include a broad range of research approaches, including qualitative studies (Stevens). These reviews undergo a rigorous peer review process to ensure they meet exacting standards, so the EBP team may rate the strength of evidence at the level of the research synthesized in the review if it is not a meta-analysis (in which case it would be Level I evidence). For example, if the Cochrane review includes quasi-experimental studies, recommendations based on this review would be considered Level II evidence, as discussed in Chapter 6.

Peer reviewed health-care journals also publish systematic reviews. The quality of these reviews is dependent on the type and quality of the primary studies evaluated. Therefore, the magnitude of evidence presented in systematic reviews would be directly proportional to the level of evidence in the primary studies reviewed. Reports of primary research included in non-peer reviewed systematic reviews should be appraised before rating the strength of evidence at the research level. Otherwise, the EBP team should interpret non-peer reviewed systematic reviews as level IV evidence.

Clinical Practice Guidelines (Level IV Evidence)

Despite efforts to ensure quality, the degree to which clinical practice guidelines (CPGs) draw from existing evidence can fluctuate. Most guidelines are based on systematic reviews, developed by experts whose charge is to arrive at specific clinical conclusions (Institute of Medicine, 2001). The evidence base can be limited or conflicting—judgment exercised when arriving at recommendations. Additionally, guidelines can lack the specificity needed to ensure consistent application across patients with the same clinical situation. Therefore, as with other summative research reviews, the strength and quality of guideline recommendations (Level IV) are a product of the supporting evidence's type and quality (Dykes, 2003).

In response to concerns about the methodological quality of CPGs, an international collaboration developed the AGREE Instrument, a 23-item assessment divided into six independent domains (AGREE, 2005). Key identifiers of CPG quality are scope and purpose, stakeholder involvement, rigor of development, clarity and presentation, applicability, and editorial independence (Wimpenny, 2007).

Recently, there has been attention paid to assessing equity in clinical practice guidelines. Equity concerns arise in groups potentially vulnerable to inequity because of residence, race, occupation, gender, religion, education, socioeconomic status, social network, and capital (Dans et al., 2007). When appropriate, an EBP team will need to consider the sociopolitical dimensions of applying CPGs to disadvantaged patient populations.

The age of the patient population is equally important. Consider the anatomic, physiologic, and developmental differences between children and adults before applying published guidelines. For example, Baharestani and Ratliff (2007) noted that many pressure ulcer prevention protocols for neonates and children have been extrapolated from adult practice guidelines, raising concerns about whether the needs of pediatric patients at risk for pressure ulcer have been adequately addressed.

It is important to note that although groups of experts create these guidelines, which frequently carry a professional society's seal of approval, opinions that convert data to recommendations require subjective judgments that in turn leave room for error and bias (Detsky, 2006). Potential conflicts of interest can be generated by financial interests, job description, personal research interests, and previous experience. An awareness of bias potential is essential when appraising the quality of CPGs.

Expert Opinion

The previous sections on summative publications represent the opinions of recognized experts on research-based evidence. Often an EBP team uncovers opinions (published and otherwise) on non-research–based evidence. Expert opinions are revealed in published case studies, narrative literature reviews (previously contrasted to systematic reviews), or written and spoken advice of a recognized expert with extensive clinical experience and expertise.

Case Studies (Level V Evidence)

A *case study* (Level V) is an in-depth look at a single person, group, or other social unit to obtain a wealth of descriptive information in order to attempt to understand issues important to the phenomenon under study (Polit & Beck, 2004). It can be quantitative or qualitative in nature. Although some publications are titled case *studies*, often they are case *reports*, presenting a summary of anecdotal descriptions of a particular patient care scenario. True case studies require the following design elements: research question(s), propositions, unit of analysis, logic linking the data to its propositions, and criteria for interpreting findings (Yin, 1994). There are also three approaches, or *intents*, to case study design: *exploratory, explanatory,* and *descriptive* (Zucker, 2001).

An example of a *case report* that purports to be a *case study* is *"Aortic Aneurysm in Pregnancy: A Case Study"* (Robinson, 2005), which contains details on a single patient (pathophysiology, patient presentation, assessment, and nursing interventions) but fails to provide any of Yin's essential elements. An example of rigorous use of case study methodology is *"Direct Care Workers' Response to Dying and Death in the Nursing Home: A Case Study"* (Black & Rubenstein, 2004), which describes a substudy of a multiyear, multisite ethnographic study that used interviews, informal conversations, and on-site observations.

Narrative Literature Reviews (Level V Evidence)

As stated previously, traditional narrative reviews abound in the literature. Traditional literature reviews are not confined to summaries of scientific literature; they can also present a narrative description of information from non-scientific literature, including reports of organizational experience and opinions of experts. Such reviews possess some of the desired attributes of a systematic review, but not the same standardized approach, appraisal, and critical review of the studies. For example, an author of a narrative review of research studies related to a particular question may describe comprehensive, even replicable, literature search strategies but neglect to appraise the quality of the studies discussed.

An example of a narrative literature review is "The Forensic Mental Health Nurse: A Literature Review" (Bowring-Lossock, 2006), which draws information from published studies as well as reports of competencies, knowledge, and skills required by forensic mental health nurses.

Advice of Individual Experts (Level V Evidence)

The opinions of experts take the form of commentary articles, position statements, case reports, or letters to the editor. Expert opinion may also be written and verbal communication with a recognized expert. Outside recognition that a professional is an expert is critical to determining the confidence an EBP team has in the expert's recommendations. The expertise of an author of commentaries and opinion pieces can be difficult to discern. In addition to perusing an author's education, work, and university affiliations, an EBP team can check whether the author has published extensively on the topic, others have cited the author's work, or the author is a recognized speaker.

Organizational Experience

Reports of organizational experience often take the form of quality improvement reports, financial data, and program evaluations. These sources of evidence can be internal to an EBP team's organization or published reports from external organizations.

Quality Improvement Reports (Level V Evidence)

Because testing interventions through randomized controlled trials is not always possible with patients who have multiple chronic conditions, lessons learned from continuous quality improvement (QI) initiatives provide an EBP team with another source of evidence (Level V; Vratny & Shriver, 2007). The organizational experience described here is distinctly different from organizational improvement, quality-focused research, or health-services research intended to generalize results. Health-services research uses experimental, quasi-experimental, or non-experimental research designs (described in Chapter 6) and should be reviewed and appraised as such.

QI is a method of self-examination to inform improvement efforts at the local level. During its review of non-research evidence, an EBP team should examine internal QI data relating to the practice question as well as QI initiatives based on similar questions published by peer institutions. While organizations become more mature in their QI efforts, they become more rigorous in the approach, the analysis of results, and the use of established measures as metrics (Newhouse, Pettit, Poe, & Rocco, 2006). In contrast to research studies, the findings from quality improvement studies are not meant to be generalized to other settings. Organizations that may benefit from the findings need to make decisions regarding implementation based on the characteristics of their organization.

QI reporting is an internal process; nevertheless, the desire to share the results from such projects is evident in the growing number of collaborative efforts targeting particular risk-prone issues. For example, The Institute of Healthcare Improvement (IHI) sponsors the IMPACT Network (IHI, 2007), a learning and innovation network of quality-focused organizations working together to achieve improvement in health-care areas, such as perinatal care and reducing surgical complications. Results of these activities are presented at conferences and seminars, providing others the opportunity to learn about the latest improvement ideas. Although evidence obtained from QI initiatives is not as strong as that obtained through scientific inquiry, the sharing of successful QI stories has the potential to identify future EBP questions, QI projects, or research studies external to the organization.

An example of how a quality improvement collaborative translates prevention into clinical practice using facility reports and chart abstraction is "Translating Evidence-Based Falls Prevention Into Clinical Practice in Nursing Facilities: Results and Lessons From a Quality Improvement Collaborative" (Colón-Emeric et al., 2006).

Financial Data (Level V Evidence)

The EBP team will find research studies of cost-effectiveness and economic evaluations in the literature. For example, on reading a report on a study that compared the profitability ratios between matched pairs of ANCC Magnet-designated and non-Magnet facilities using financial statements for 2 fiscal years (Tauzon, 2007), the EBP team would discover that this was actually a descriptive, non-experimental design research study using comparative data analysis between two groups of facilities. Therefore, the strength and quality of evidence obtained from this study would be judged using criteria identified in Chapter 6 on appraising research evidence.

An EBP team can find reports of cost-effectiveness and economic evaluations that do *not* fall within the realm of research (Level V) in published data or from internal organizational reports. An *economic evaluation* applies analytic techniques to identify, measure, and compare the costs and outcomes of two or more alternative programs or interventions (Centers for Disease Control and Prevention, 2007). A common economic evaluation of health-care decision making is a *cost-effectiveness analysis*, which compares costs of alternative interventions that produce a common health outcome. Although results of such an analysis can provide justification for a program, empirical evidence can provide support for an increase in program funding or a switch from one program to another (Centers for Disease Control and Prevention, 2007). Anderson et al. (2003) provides other economic evaluations:

- *cost-analysis:* the systematic collection, categorization, and analysis of all resources consumed by a health intervention or program

- *cost-benefit:* converts all costs and benefits of a program into dollars, allowing comparison of programs that have disparate outcomes

- *cost-utility:* a special variant of cost-effectiveness analysis that allows for the comparison of programs that address different health problems (e.g., breast cancer screening and diabetes control, because the outcomes are converted into a common health metric, such as quality-adjusted life years)

Carande-Kulis et al. (2000) suggested standard inclusion criteria for economic studies consist of an analytic method (such as one previously mentioned) and provide sufficient detail regarding the method and results. In assessing the quality of the economic study, the Community Guide's Economic Evaluation Abstraction Form (2001) suggests that the following questions be asked: Was the study population well-described? Was the question being analyzed well-defined? Did the study define the time frame? Were data sources for all costs reported? Were data sources and costs appropriate with respect to the program and population being tested? Was the primary outcome measure clearly specified? Did outcomes include the effects or unintended outcomes of the program? Was the analytic model reported in an explicit manner? Were sensitivity analyses performed?

An example of an economic study of a non-research nature is "Cost and Clinical Outcomes of a Back Clinic" (New & Winecoff, 2007), which analyzed the financial impact of a back clinic on a single health-care facility using organizational occupational health and human resource data.

Program Evaluations (Level V Evidence)

Internal and external program evaluations can provide another glimpse at non-research evidence. Although program evaluations may be conducted within a framework of scientific inquiry and designed as research studies, most internal program evaluations are less rigorous (Level V). Frequently, there will be pre- and post-implementation data at the organizational level, accompanied by qualitative reports of personal satisfaction with the program.

Program evaluations are often conducted under formative or summative organizational assessments or a quality improvement umbrella. An example of a program evaluation is "*Implementation and Evaluation of a Nursing Home Fall Management Program* (Rask et al., 2007), which collected information on process-of-care documentation and fall and physical restraint use rates derived from quality improvement activities.

Practitioner Experience and Expertise

The concept of holistic care as the hallmark of nursing expertise as advocated by Benner (2001) supports the notion that evidence of all types (both research and non-research) must inform nursing practice. Novice nurses rely heavily on guidelines and care protocols to enhance skill development, looking at the patient as the sum of composite parts. The more experienced expert nurse has gained an intuitive grasp of each clinical situation and looks at each aspect of care as it pertains to the whole patient (Christensen & Hewitt-Taylor, 2006).

Practitioner expertise (Level V), both skill proficiency and professional judgment, is gained through a combination of education and clinical experiences. Personal judgments arising from past and present nurse-patient interactions and knowledge about what works within the organization or system add depth to that expertise. Nurses who practice within an evidence-based framework are committed to personal growth, reflection, self-evaluation, accountability, and lifelong learning (Dale, 2006).

"The Expertise in Practice Project" (Hardy, Titchen, Manley, & McCormack, 2006) in the United Kingdom identified and examined attributes of nurse expertise as well as enabling factors. Identified attributes of expertise included:

- *holistic practice knowledge:* drawing from a range of knowledge bases to inform action

- *skilled know-how:* enabling others by sharing knowledge and skills

- *saliency:* observing non-verbal cues to understand each individual's unique situation

- *moral agency:* consciously promoting each individual's dignity, respect, and individuality

- *knowing the patient/client:* promoting patient decision making within the context of each individual's unique perspective

Enabling factors for nursing expertise included *reflectivity* (the ability to continually reconsider, reassess, and reframe one's work), *organization of practice* (organization and prioritization of workload), *autonomy and authority*, *good interpersonal relationships*, and *recognition from others*.

Although this book provides a model and guidelines to increase a nurse's expertise in evidence-based care, the best application of EBP occurs within the interdisciplinary care team, because no one discipline provides health care in isolation. Dale (2006) suggests guidelines and principles for EBP that include (1) the team's collective responsibility for the quality of the patient's experience and subsequent health outcomes, (2) each practitioner's accountability to his or her profession, (3) each practitioner's responsibility to exercise clinical judgment judiciously when determining the evidence that will best inform care, and (4) the team's collective responsibility to ensure that patients are involved in decision-making processes throughout the continuum of care.

Patient Experience (Level 5 Evidence)

The art of nursing recognizes that humans are "intentional, free beings who actively participate in their life and choose ways of becoming" (Milton, 2007, p. 125). Health is a quality of life and is best described by the person who is experiencing it. Patient experience (Level V) is a core component of a patient-centered approach to care, honoring humanly lived experiences as evidence in order for the patient to be an active partner in decision making. This is based on the core ethical value of respect for people. Each patient has personal, religious, and cultural beliefs that influence him or her when making informed care decisions. Individuals and families of different cultures, races, and social and economic classes are likely to have very dissimilar experiences with the health-care system and, hence, have dissimilar perspectives on evidence-based practices (Birkel, Hall, Lane, Cohan, & Miller, 2003).

The expert nurse incorporates patient preferences into clinical decision making by asking the following questions: Are the research findings and non-research evidence relevant to this particular patient's care? Have all care and treatment options based on the best available evidence been presented to the patient? Has the patient been given as much time as is necessary to allow for clarification and consideration of options? Have the patient's expressed preferences and concerns been considered when planning care? The answer to these questions requires ethical practice and respect for a patient's autonomy. Combining sensitivity to individual patient needs and thoughtful application of best evidence leads to optimal patient-centered outcomes.

In this era of consumer-driven health care, nurses are increasingly cognizant of the critical role the consumer plays in the quality and safety of health care. Upholding the belief that consumer preferences and values are integral to EBP, Melnyk and Fineout-Overholt (2006) offered three suggestions to involve patients in clinical decision making: (1) respect patient participation in clinical decision making, (2) assess patient preferences and values during the admission intake process, and (3) provide patient education about treatment plan options. Additionally, it is important to provide information to patients about best practice recommendations, as these apply to their particular clinical situation. Only an informed patient can truly participate in clinical decision making, ensuring the best possible outcomes of care.

Engaging consumers of health care in EBP goes well beyond the individual patient encounter. Consumer organizations can play a significant role in supporting implementation and promulgation of EBP. Consumer-led activities can take the form of facilitating research to expedite equitable adoption of new and existing best practices, promoting policies for the development and use of advocacy toolkits, and influencing provider adoption of EBP (Birkel, Hall, Lane, Cohan, & Miller 2003). An EBP team should take into consideration the perspectives of children, young families, the elderly, and aging families. They should ascertain whether suggested recommendations have been designed and developed with sensitivity and knowledge of diverse cultural groups.

Appraising the Quality of Non-Research Evidence

Appendix G presents the JHNEBP Non-research Evidence Appraisal, developed for nurses to use when appraising the strength and quality of recommendations found in non-research evidence. The goal of this tool is to capture on one page the standard questions that guide an EBP team in determining the strength of the recommendations and the quality of non-research evidence. The EBP team judges the relevance of the particular question's evidence as well as the clarity of the recommendations. Additional questions are divided into four sections: systematic reviews, clinical practice guidelines, organizational data, and expert opinion.

The first section lists questions pertinent to the appraisal of systematic reviews. An emphasis is placed on the comprehensiveness of search strategies—the criteria used to determine which studies were reviewed, the presentation of the relevant details of each study, the disclosure of methodological limitations, and the appropriateness of the selected studies. Evidence from a systematic review is lower in strength (Level IV) than evidence from individual studies that may have been included in the review. True evidential strength comes from the primary studies in the review, not the review itself, because a systematic review is a secondary source and is subject to reviewer bias. The valuable, well-executed systematic review identifies primary studies that are worth further review by an EBP team.

The second section's questions help evaluate the strength and quality of recommendations made in the clinical practice guidelines. Here, an EBP team ascertains the source and rigor of the guidelines, target populations of the guidelines, potential biases, and clarity of recommendations. As with evidence obtained in the systematic review, an EBP team should seek primary studies to determine the strength of evidence of individual guideline recommendations.

Questions listed in the third section frame the organizational data, emphasizing the importance of clear aims, methods, metrics, analytic procedures, and interpretations. Special attention is paid to making sure that the setting in which data were gathered is similar to the setting of interest to the EBP team.

Questions in the final section appraise evidence from expert opinion. These questions force the team to look for evidence of expertise and to determine whether this expertise lies in a single individual or in a collective group. The team makes a judgment as to whether the opinions are research-based evidence, non-research–based evidence, or a combination.

The second page of the tool contains descriptors of non-research reviews, differentiating Level IV evidential strength (supported by research evidence) and Level V evidential strength (supported by non-research evidence). A quality grid for both summative reviews and expert opinions, tailored to capture desired elements of each, is listed in Table 7.1.

Appendix H and Appendix I can assist an EBP team in summarizing non-research evidence. This structured approach to combining the outcomes of the EBP team's review of both research and non-research evidence allows for a holistic approach in the development of recommendations for change.

Recommendations for Nurse Leaders

Time and resource constraints compel nurse leaders to find creative ways to support integration of new knowledge into clinical practice. The time that the average staff nurse has to devote to gathering and appraising evidence is limited. Therefore, finding the most efficient way to gain new knowledge should be a goal of EBP initiatives (Chapter 9 suggests ways to build organizational EBP infrastructure). Summative research reviews provide a completed summation of evidence related to a specific practice question. If a systematic review that relates to the practice question and setting of interest is already complete, additional critical review of evidence may not be required. Ensuring that nurses have the skills required to critically appraise recommendations put forth in summative research reviews will serve to streamline time spent in EBP activities related to a given practice question. Nurse leaders should not only support staff education initiatives that teach nurses how to read and interpret summative research reviews, but they should also become familiar with desired attributes of such reviews so that they serve as credible mentors in the change process.

The challenge to the nurse is to combine the contributions of the two evidence types (research and non-research) in making patient-care decisions. According to Melnyk and Fineout-Overholt (2006), there is no "magic bullet" or standard formula with which to determine how much weight should be applied to each of these factors when making patient-care decisions. It is not sufficient to apply a standard rating system that grades the strength and quality of evidence without determining whether recommendations made by the best evidence are compatible with the patient's values and preferences and the clinician's expertise. Nurse leaders can best support EBP by providing clinicians with the knowledge and skills necessary to appraise quantitative and qualitative research evidence within the context of non-research evidence. Only through continual learning can clinicians gain the confidence needed to incorporate the broad range of evidence into the more targeted care of individual patients.

References

Agency for Healthcare Research and Quality. (2007, September). *Evidence-based practice centers*. Retrieved September 1, 2006, from http://www.ahrq.gov/clinic/epc

The AGREE Research Trust. (2005). *The AGREE Instrument*. Retrieved October 20, 2007, from http://www.agreetrust.org/instrument.htm

Alderson, P., Green, S., & Higgins, J P. (Eds.). (2005). *Cochrane Library, Issue 1*. Chichester, UK: Wiley.

Anderson, L. M., Fielding, J. E., Fullilove, M. T., Scrimshaw, S. C., Carande-Sulis, V. G., & Task Force on Community Preventive Services. (2003). Methods for conducting systematic reviews of the evidence of effectiveness and economic efficiency of interventions to promote healthy social environments. *American Journal of Preventive Medicine, 24*(3, Suppl 1.), 25-31.

Baharestani, M. M., & Ratliff, C. T. (2007). Pressure ulcers in neonates and children: A NPUAP white paper. *Advances in Skin & Wound Care, 20*(4), 208, 210, 212, 214, 216, 218-220.

Benner, P. E. (2001). *From novice to expert: Excellence and power in clinical nursing practice. Commemorative edition.* Upper Saddle River, NJ: Prentice Hall.

Birkel, R. C., Hall, L. L., Lane, T., Cohan, K., & Miller, J. (2003). Consumers and families as partners in implementing evidence-based practice. *Psychiatric Clinics of North America, 26,* 867-881.

Black, H. K., & Rubenstein, R. L. (2005). Direct care workers' response to dying and death in the nursing home: A case study. *The Journals of Gerontology Series B: Psychological Sciences and Social Sciences, 60,* S3-S10.

Bowring-Lossock, E. (2006). The forensic mental health nurse—a literature review. *Journal of Psychiatric and Mental Health Nursing, 13*(6), 780-785.

Carande-Kulis, V. G., Maciosek, M. V., Briss, P. A., Teutsch, S. M., Zaza, S., Truman, B. I., et al. & Task Force on Community Preventive Services. (2003). Methods for systematic reviews of economic evaluations. *American Journal of Preventive Medicine, 18*(1S), 75-91.

Carper, B. (1978). Fundamental patterns of knowing in nursing. *ANS. Advances in Nursing Science, 1*(1), 13-23.

Centers for Disease Control and Prevention. (2007). Economic evaluation of public health preparedness and response efforts. Retrieved August 4, 2007, from http://www.cdc.gov/owcd/EET/SeriesIntroduction/TOC.html

Christensen, M., & Hewitt-Taylor, J. (2006). From expert to task, expert nursing practice redefined? *Journal of Clinical Nursing, 15*(12), 1531-1539.

Ciliska, D., Cullum, N., & Marks, S. (2001). Evaluation of systematic reviews of treatment or prevention interventions. *Evidence-Based Nursing, 4,* 100-104.

The Cochrane Collaboration. (2006, September). *Cochrane Reviewer's Handbook.* Retrieved October 20, 2007, from http://www.cochrane.org/resources/handbook/

Colón-Emeric, C., Schenck, A., Gorospe, J., McArdle, J., Dobson, L., DePorter, C., & McConnell, E. (2006). Translating evidence-based falls prevention into clinical practice in nursing facilities: Results and lessons from a quality improvement collaborative. *American Journal of Geriatrics Society, 54,* 1414-1418.

Community Guide Economic Evaluation Abstraction, Version 3.0. (2001). Retrieved August 12, 2007, from www.thecommunityguide.org/methods/econ-abs-form.pdf

Conn, V.S. (2004). Meta-analysis research. *Journal of Vascular Nursing, 22*(2), 51-52.

Dale, A. E. (2006). Determining guiding principles for evidence-based practice. *Nursing Standard, 20*(25), 41-46.

Dans, A. M., Dans, L., Oxman, A. D., Robinson, V., Acuin, J., Tugwell, P., et al. (2007). Assessing equity in clinical practice guidelines. *Journal of Clinical Epidemiology, 60*, 540-546.

Detsky, A. S. (2006). Sources of bias for authors of clinical practice guidelines. *Canadian Medical Association Journal, 175*(9), 1033.

Dykes, P. C. (2003). Practice guidelines and measurement: state of the science. *Nursing Outlook, 51*(2), 65-69.

Fervers, B., Burgers, J. S., Haugh, M. C., Brouwers, M., Browman, G., Luzeau, F., et al. (2005, January 21). Predictors of high quality clinical practice guidelines: Examples in oncology. *International Journal for Quality in Health Care Advance Access*, 1-10.

Gage, J. D., Everett, K. D., & Bullock, L. (2006). Integrative review of parenting in nursing research. *Journal of Nursing Scholarship, 38*, 58-62.

Green, S., & Higgins, J. (Eds.). (2005). Glossary. Cochrane handbook for systematic reviews of interventions 4.2.5. Retrieved September 1, 2006, from http://www.cochrane.dk/cochrane/handbook/handbook.htm

Hardy, S., Titchen, A., Manley, K., & McCormack, B. (2006). Re-defining nursing expertise in the United Kingdom. *Nursing Science Quarterly, 19*, 260-264.

Hines, P. S., Gattuso, J. S., Barnwell, E., Cofer, M., Kellum, L., Mattox, S., et al. (2003). Translating psychosocial research findings into practice guidelines. *Journal of Nursing Administration, 33*(7/8), 397-403.

Institute of Healthcare Improvement. (n.d.). *IMPACT improvement/action.* Retrieved October 21, 2007, from http://www.ihi.org/IHI/Programs/ IMPACTNetwork/

Institute of Medicine. (2001). *Crossing the quality chasm. A new health system for the 21st century.* Washington DC: National Academy Press.

Institute of Medicine, Field, M. J., & Lohr, K. N. (Eds.). (1992). *Guidelines for clinical practice: From development to use.* Washington, DC: National Academy Press.

Kent, B., & Fineout-Overholt, E. (2007). Teaching EBP: Part 1. Making sense of clinical practice guidelines. *Worldviews on Evidence-Based Nursing, 4*(2), 106-111.

Melnyk, B. M., & Fineout-Overholt, E. (2006). Consumer preferences and values as an integral key to evidence-based practice. *Nursing Administration Quarterly, 30*(2), 123-127.

Milton, C. (2007). Evidence-based practice: Ethical questions for nursing. *Nursing Science Quarterly, 20*(2), 123-126.

Mosca, L., Appel, L. J., Benjamin, E. J., Berra, K., Chandra-Strobos, N., Fabunmi, et al. (2004). Evidence-based guidelines for cardiovascular disease prevention in women. *Circulation, 109*(5), 672-693.

National Guideline Clearinghouse. (2005). Criteria for inclusion of clinical practice guidelines in NGC. Retrieved September 1, 2006, from www.guidelines.gov

New, F. R., & Winecoff, A. (2007). Cost and clinical outcomes of a back injury clinic. *Nursing Economic$, 25*(2), 127-129.

Newhouse, R. P., Pettit, J. C., Poe, S., & Rocco, L. (2006). The slippery slope: differentiating between quality improvement and research. *Journal of Nursing Administration, 36*(4), 211-219.

Polit, D. F., & Beck, C. T. (2004). *Nursing research: Principles and methods* (7th ed.). Philadelphia: Lippincott Williams & Wilkens.

Popay, J. (2006). *The Cochrane Qualitative Methods Group.* Retrieved September 1, 2006, from http://www.mrw.interscience.wiley.com/cochrane/clabout/articles/ CE000142/frame.html

Rask, K., Parmalee, P. A., Taylor, J. A., Green, D., Brown, H., Hawley, J., et al. (2007). Implementation and evaluation of a nursing home fall management program. *Journal of the American Geriatric Society, 55*(3), 464-466.

Robinson, R. (2005). Aortic aneurysm in pregnancy: A case study. *Dimensions in Critical Care Nursing, 24,* 21-24.

Schmid, A., Hoffman, L., Happ, M., Wolf, G. A., & DeVita, M. (2007). Failure to rescue: A literature review. *Journal of Nursing Administration, 37*(4), 188-198.

Shiffman, R. N., Shekelle, P., Overhage, M., Slutsky, J., Grimshaw, J., & Aniruddha, M. D. (2003). Standardized reporting of clinical practice guidelines: A proposal from the conference on guideline standardization. *Annals of Internal Medicine, 139,* 493-498.

Stetler, C. B., Morsi, D., Rucki, S., Broughton, S., Corrigan, B., Fitzgerald, J., et al. (1998). Utilization-focused integrative reviews in a nursing service. *Applied Nursing Research, 11*(4), 195-206.

Stevens, K. R. (2002). The truth about EBP and RCTs. *Journal of Nursing Administration, 32*(5), 232-233.

Tauzon, N. (2007) Is magnet a money-maker? *Nursing Management, 38*(6), 24, 26, 28-30.

Vratny, A., & Shriver, D. (2007). A conceptual model for growing evidence-based practice. *Nursing Administration Quarterly, 31*(2), 162-170.

Whittemore, R. (2005). Combining evidence in nursing research: Methods and implications. *Nursing Research, 54*(1), 56-62.

Wimpenny, P. (2007). Appraising and comparing pressure ulcer guidelines. *Worldviews on Evidence-Based Nursing, 4*(1), 40-50.

Yin, R. K. (1994). *Case study research: Design and methods* (2nd ed.). Newbury Park, CA: Sage.

Zucker, D. M. (2001). Using case study methodology in nursing research. *The Qualitative Report, 6*(2), 1-12. Retrieved August 20, 2006, from http://www.nova.edu/ssss/QR/QR6-2/zucker.html

Other Resources

Barbour, R. S., & Barbour, M. (2003). Evaluating and synthesizing qualitative research: the need to develop a distinctive approach. *Journal of Evaluation in Clinical Practice, 9*(2), 179-186.

Beck, C. T. (2003). Seeing the forest for the trees: A qualitative synthesis project. *Journal of Nursing Education, 42*(7), 318-323.

Dixon-Woods, M., Agarwal, S., Jones, D., Young, B., & Sutton, A. (2005). Synthesizing qualitative and quantitative evidence: A review of possible methods. *Journal of Health Services Research & Policy, 10*(1), 45-53.

Ferguson, L. M., & Day, R. A. (2004). Supporting new nurses in evidence-based practice. *Journal of Nursing Administration, 34*(11), 490-492.

Holmes, S. B., & Brown, S. J. (2005). Skeletal pin site care: National Association of Orthopaedic Nurses guidelines for orthopaedic nursing. *Orthopaedic Nursing, 24*, 99-107.

Jones, M. L. (2004). Application of systematic review methods to qualitative research: Practical issues. *Journal of Advanced Nursing, 48*(3), 271-278.

Jones, M. L. (2005). Role development and effective practice in specialist and advanced practice roles in acute hospital settings: Systematic review and meta-synthesis. *Journal of Advanced Nursing, 49*(2), 191-209.

Pancorbo-Hildalgo, P. L., Garcia-Fernandez, F. P., Lopez-Medina, I. M., & Alvarez-Nieto, C. (2006). Risk assessment scales for pressure ulcer prevention: a systematic review. *Journal of Advanced Nursing, 54*, 94-110.

Reddy, M., Gill, S. S., & Rochon, P. A. (2006). Preventing pressure ulcers: a systematic review. *JAMA, 296*, 974-984.

Sandelowski, M., Docherty, S., & Emden, C. (1997). Qualitative metasynthesis: Issues and techniques. *Research in Nursing & Health, 20*, 365-371.

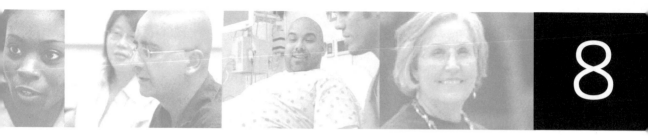

Translation

The final step of the PET process is *translation*, which assesses the evidence-based recommendations identified in the evidence phase for transferability to the setting. If appropriate, the practices are implemented, evaluated, and communicated within and outside the organization. It is the value-added step in evidence-based practice, leading to a change in nursing processes and resulting outcomes.

This chapter covers the translation phase of PET, ranging from the practice decision through dissemination. The chapter's objectives are to

- discuss criteria that determine recommendation implementation
- distinguish among PET, EBP, research, and QI
- describe the components of an action plan
- identify steps in implementing change
- discuss potential forums for communicating results

Translation is the primary reason to conduct an evidence-based review. Particular attention to planning the implementation of recommendations can improve the potential for successfully meeting the project's goals. Additionally, fully realized translation requires organizational support, human and material resources, and a commitment of individuals and interdisciplinary teams.

Critically appraising, rating, and grading the evidence and making practice recommendations require one set of skills; translation requires another. Change theory, motivational theory, political savvy, organizational processes, and dynamics of power all flourish within translation, where a number of steps occur:

- assess the feasibility and appropriateness of the recommendation

- create an action plan

- pilot (small-scale implementation) and evaluate the change

- report to appropriate channel(s)

- foster support

- create a plan for wider implementation

- communicate findings

The first step in translation is asking this question: Should we implement this practice recommendation? The JHNEBP Project Management Tool (Appendix E) is available to guide the translation process.

Criteria for Recommendation Support

Although evidence-based practice (EBP) recommendations made in the evidence phase are based on strong evidence, not all recommendations can be implemented in all settings. The use of recommendations adoption criteria helps to determine whether they are feasible in the specific practice setting. The main question is: Is this practice change implementable, given the current organizational infrastructure? What additional action or resources are needed?

Stetler (2001) recommends using the criteria of *substantiating evidence*, *fit of setting*, *feasibility*, and *current practice*. When considering the overall evidence summary, consider the finding's *consistency* (were results the same in evidence reviewed), *quality* (extent to which bias was minimized in individual studies), and *quantity* (number, sample size and power, and size of effect; Agency for Healthcare Research and Quality, 2002). Organizational context and infrastructure, such as resources (equipment or products), change agency, and organizational readiness, also need consideration (Greenhalgh, Robert, Macfarlane, Bate, & Kyriakidou, 2004). Additionally, nursing related factors, such as nursing processes, policies, and competencies, need to be present before implementing recommendations. The following guiding questions can help to determine if the proposed recommendation adds value:

- Would this change improve clinical outcomes?

- Would this change improve patient or nurse satisfaction?

- Would this change reduce the cost of care for patients?

- Would this change improve unit operations?

Determining the feasibility of implementing EBP recommendations is important in assessing whether recommendations significantly add to improving a specific problem. Implementing processes with a low likelihood of success wastes valuable time and resources on efforts that produce negligible benefits.

Possible Choices: EBP, Research, and QI

Often, problems that do not have a clear recommendation exist because of a lack of evidence, conflicting results, or a need for application to a new population or setting of interest. Some teams rely on consensus or expert agreement to make a recommendation, noting the low evidence rating. Others conduct research to test a new procedure or product.

Although beyond the scope of this chapter, research requires additional organizational infrastructure, including affiliation with an institutional review board (RB), experienced mentors who can serve as principal investigators, education in human subject research, and a number of additional research competencies. However, it is important to clearly distinguish among the activities of research, quality improvement (QI), and EBP (Newhouse, 2007b; Newhouse, Pettit, Rocco, & Poe, 2006). Box 8.1 describes the common definitions and provides an example of each.

Box 8.1.

EBP, Quality Improvement, and Research

EBP Example

This book focuses on EBP and the Practice question, Evidence, and Translation process (PET). The PET process is used to make a decision when a significant clinical, administrative, or education problem arises that requires a critical review of scientific and non-scientific evidence. The evidence is summarized using a rating scale, recommendations are made based on the evidence, and recommendations are implemented and evaluated. The PET process uses the organization's quality improvement (QI) program to implement and evaluate recommendations.

EBP Example: For adult patients admitted with heart failure, what is the best education strategy for an improved smoking cessation attempt? An evidence review is conducted using the PET process, with recommendations generated, implemented, and evaluated using the QI process.

QI Example

In QI, individuals work together for system and process improvements with the intent to improve outcomes (Committee on Assessing the System for Protecting Human Research Participants, 2002), or use a data-driven systematic approach that improves care locally (Baily, Bottrell, Lynn, & Jennings, 2006). EBP projects inform which procedures, nursing interventions, or processes to implement and evaluate.

QI Example: Standard measurement of compliance with smoking cessation counseling for patients with heart failure. Compliance with the smoking cessation standard is measured as present or absent for patients and reported for improvement purposes and public reporting.

Research Example

Research is "a systematic investigation, including research development, testing, and evaluation, designed to develop or contribute to generalizable knowledge" (Department of Health and Human Services, 2005). Examples of research include testing changes in current practice, comparing standard care with new approaches, or evaluating new health-care strategies or therapies to expand what is known (National Bioethics Commission, 2001). Research activities are intended to be generalized or applied outside of an organization and require compliance with Office for Human Research Protections (OHRP) regulations, and sometimes the Food and Drug Administration (FDA).

Research Example: A randomized controlled design is used to test whether a new nurse-intensive counseling session prior to discharge is more effective than standard teaching to improve smoking cessation attempts for patients who have a diagnosis of heart failure.

The Action Plan

Creating an action plan enables the team to provide manageable implementation steps and assign responsibility for carrying the project forward. The team now develops the specific change strategies to introduce, promote, and evaluate the recommended change. The action plan will include:

- The development of (or change to) a protocol, guideline, critical pathway, or system/process related to the EBP question;

- The specification of a detailed time line assigning team members to the tasks needed to implement the change (including the evaluation process and reporting of results); and

- The solicitation of feedback from organizational leadership, bedside clinicians, and other stakeholders on the action plan.

Considerations must include assessment of the system's readiness for change and implementation strategies targeted to overcome barriers. Readiness for change assessment will include the availability of human and material resources, current processes, support from decision makers (individuals and groups), and budget implication. Specific implementation processes will include communication pathways, the education plan and involvement of stakeholders and individuals affected. Additional detail on constructing and evaluating outcomes is included in the following section.

The action plan should be incorporated into the QI activities using organizational tools, processes, and reporting mechanisms. The Model for Improvement, developed by Associates in Process Improvement (2007), is commonly used by EBP teams in such a way. The Model for Improvement includes a process called the *Plan-Do-Study-Act* cycle (PDSA). Tips for using this process and tools are available on the Institute for Healthcare Improvement (IHI) Web site (2007a). Steps in the Model for Improvement include forming the team, setting aims, establishing measures, selecting changes, implementing changes, and spreading changes (IHI, 2007a).

It can be helpful to formulate the plan in a template that includes a time line with progress columns. Use the JHNEBP Project Management Tool (Appendix C) or similar organizational template to monitor progress.

Implementing Change

The pilot or small test of change

After creation of an action plan, the actual implementation begins. The first step is a small test of the change, or *pilot*. The implementation plan is communicated to all team members who are affected by the change or who are caring for a patient/population affected by the change. This communication can take the form of an agenda item at a staff meeting, inservice, direct mail, e-mail, bulletin board, video, and so on. Team members must know who the leader responsible for the change is and where to access needed information or supplies. Changes are then implemented and evaluated.

Change or adoption of new knowledge theories can guide and inform effective strategies to enable a successful implementation process (Rogers, 1983; Greenhalgh et al., 2004). What is known about the state of current organizational change theory can be applied to EBP initiatives (Newhouse, 2007a).

Evaluating Outcomes

After the change is implemented, the next step is to evaluate the impact of the change and the progress toward the desired outcome. Evaluation metrics consistent with organizational QI processes and tools should be used at appropriate intervals to measure the change. The major steps in selecting and developing the metrics include defining the purpose of measurement, choosing the clinical areas to evaluate, selecting the indicators, developing design specifications for the measures, and evaluating the indicators (Pronovost, Miller, Dorman, Berenholtz, & Rubin, 2001 [adapted from McGlynn, 1998]). Measures may include *process measures* (focus on steps in the system), *outcome measures* (focus on results of system performance), or *balancing measures* (focus on impact on other parts of the system; IHI, 2007b).

Data collected are compared to baseline data to determine whether the change should be implemented on a wider scale. Descriptive data, such as *frequencies* or *means*, can be graphically displayed in bar, line, or run charts.

Reporting results of preliminary evaluation to decision makers

After the outcome evaluation, a report to the appropriate committee or decision makers should follow. Decision makers can be a committee, such as a research or quality improvement committee, or organizational leaders. The report should be a succinct communication in an executive summary format consistent with organizational templates. Box 8.2 provides an example of an executive summary framed in the PET template.

Box 8.2.

Example of Template for Executive Summary Using PET

Practice question

There is an increase in the incidence of postoperative pressure ulcers. When patients are positioned in the operating room (OR), the team uses multiple positioning aids, and the protocol is not standardized. The question posed is: What are the most effective interventions to prevent skin pressure in adult patients undergoing surgery?

Evidence

CINAHL and PubMed were searched using the key words perioperative or surgery, AND positioning, AND pressure ulcers; 18 sources of evidence were reviewed.

Category Level	Number of Studies	Summary of Findings	Overall Rating
Level I	5	■ Foam is not found better than conventional nursing care. ■ Gel pads are better than standard OR mattresses.	B

Category Level	Number of Studies	Summary of Findings	Overall Rating
		■ Screening should be conducted for specific risk factors.	
		■ There is no difference between low flow pressure mattresses and alternating pressure mattresses.	
		■ Multi-cell dynamic pressure pulsating mattresses are more effective than conventional mattresses.	
Level II	4	■ Conduct screening for specific risk factors.	B
		■ Alternating pressure systems are effective.	
		■ Visco-elastic polyether is more effective than foam or gel.	
Level III	2	■ Screening should be conducted for specific risk factors.	A-B
Level IV	0		
Level V	7	■ Fluid pad reduced pressure ulcers.	B
		■ Foam overlays have the lowest pressure reduction.	
		■ Gel pads allow for some pressure reduction.	
		■ Dynamic air pressure mattresses are promising but need more research.	
		■ Foam pads are not effective in reducing capillary interface pressure because they quickly compress under heavy body areas.	
		■ Use of gel pads or similar devices over the OR bed decreases pressure at any given point by redistributing overall pressure across a larger surface area.	

Category Level	Number of Studies	Summary of Findings	Overall Rating
		■ Foam mattress overlays are effective in reducing pressure only if they are made of thick and dense foam that resists compression.	
		■ Pillows, blankets, and molded foam devices produce only a minimum of pressure reduction.	
		■ Towels and sheet rolls do not reduce pressure and may contribute to friction injuries.	

Translation

Recommendation:

■ Identify a team from the perioperative and inpatient areas to develop a comprehensive pressure ulcer prevention protocol that includes all perioperative phases (preoperatively through discharge).

■ The nurse manager of the OR will evaluate the use of current pressure relieving devices for patients at risk and report current practices and compliance to the nursing Quality Improvement Committee.

■ The OR Quality Improvement Committee will evaluate gel and alternating pressure mattresses in the OR and recommend changes if indicated to the Products Committee and OR Procedure Committee.

■ The OR Procedure Committee will review and standardize OR positioning protocols.

■ The OR Evidence-Based Practice Committee will develop a risk assessment/screening tool for patients undergoing surgery.

Building Organizational Support

Securing support from decision makers is critical to implementation of recommendations. Allocation of human and material resources is dependent on the endorsement of leaders or committees as well as collaboration with those individuals or groups affected by the recommendations. Human and material resources necessary to support the change should be estimated and budgeted, and an implementation plan formulated. Decision makers may support wide implementation of the change, request another small test of the change to validate results, revise the plan or recommendations, or reject the implementation plan.

Preparing for the presentation or meeting with decision makers, involving stakeholders, and creating a comprehensive implementation plan are key steps in building organizational support.

Next Steps

After favorable evaluation of the implementation of recommendations and support from decision makers, the changes are implemented on a wider scale if appropriate. The team reviews the process and results and considers the next steps. Organizational or additional unit implementation requires a modified action plan and possibly redesignation of responsibility to an individual or team with the target scope of responsibility.

New considerations for the team can include a new question that emerges from the process, additional training or education for colleagues in the process changes, and suggestions for new measures or tools for the evaluation. The recommendations are then implemented and evaluated organizationally.

Communicating Findings

The level of communication regarding the findings and dissemination of information is a factor of the problem's scope. Evidence-based project outcomes are communicated internally to all members involved in the care of the patient or population affected by the practice changes. This communication can take the form of internal meetings, committees, or conferences. Additionally, it may be appropriate to present results at professional conferences or in suitable EBP publications, sharing lessons learned, what worked, what did not, the resulting clinical and fiscal outcomes, and so on. Methods of external dissemination may also include podium or poster presentations to organizations or publication in quality journals or electronic media.

Specific guidance on how to get started with developing abstracts, presentations, and publications is available (Krenzischek & Newhouse, 2005). Local, national, and international professional organizations or university conferences are an excellent way to gain oral or poster presentation experience. See Table 8.2 for links to general and specialty organization Web sites. Search each Web site for appropriate conferences, dates, and locations. Announcements of upcoming conferences generally include information about calls for abstracts. A call for conference abstracts can be communicated via group e-mail or mail, or posted on an organization's intranet. Each abstract has specific instructions for content, length, and responsibilities.

Table 8.2.   Web Sites for Potential Conferences to Present EBP Projects

Sigma Theta Tau International:
www.nursingsociety.org
American Nurses Association General Nursing Practice Links:
www.nursingworld.org/EspeciallyForYou/Links/GeneralNursingPractice.aspx
American Nurses Association Specialty Nursing Practice Links:
www.nursingworld.org/EspeciallyForYou/Links/SpecialtyNursing.aspx
American Nurses Credentialing Centers' National Magnet Conference:
www.nursecredentialing.org/magnet/confredirect.html

Many professional nursing and multidisciplinary journals and newsletters publish manuscripts about EBP projects as articles. Author guidelines are usually available via the Internet for review. *Worldviews on Evidence-Based Nursing* focuses specifically on EBP and is an excellent resource for a potential publication.

Summary

Translation is the essence of the evidence-based practice process and the cornerstone of best practice. The organizational infrastructure needed to foster translation includes budgetary support, human and material resources, and commitment of individuals and interdisciplinary teams. Translation is the outcome of the PET process. The PET process is constructed as a linear process, but there are many steps that can generate new questions, recommendations, or actions. Translation of recommendations requires organizational skills, project management, and a leader with a high level of influence and tenacity—the perfect job for nurses.

References

Agency for Healthcare Research and Quality. (2002). Systems to rate the strength of scientific evidence. Summary. *Evidence Report/Technology Assessment: Number 47* (Rep. No. 02-E015). Rockville, MD. Retrieved August 17, 2007, from http://www.ahrq.gov/clinic/epcsums/strengthsum.htm.

Associates in Process Improvement. (2007). *Model for improvement.* Retrieved August 18, 2007, from http://www.apiweb.org/API_home_page.htm

Baily, M. A., Bottrell, M., Lynn, J., & Jennings, B. (2006). *The ethics of using QI methods to improve health care quality and safety: A Hastings Center Special Report.* Garrison, NY: The Hastings Center.

Committee on Assessing the System for Protecting Human Research Participants. (2002). *Responsible research: A systems approach to protecting research participants.* Washington, DC: The National Academies Press.

Department of Health and Human Services. (2005). *Code of Federal Regulations, 45CFR46.210.* Retrieved October 19, 2007, from http://stemcells.nih.gov/staticresources/news/newsArchives/45.htm

Greenhalgh, T., Robert, G., Macfarlane, F., Bate, P., & Kyriakidou, O. (2004). Diffusion of innovations in service organizations: Systematic review and recommendations. *Milbank Quarterly, 82,* 581-629.

Institute for Healthcare Improvement. (2007a). *How to improve.* Retrieved August 17, 2007, from http://www.ihi.org/IHI/Topics/CriticalCare/IntensiveCare/HowToImprove/

Institute for Healthcare Improvement. (2007b). *Measures.* Retrieved August 17, 2007, from http://www.ihi.org/IHI/Topics/Improvement/ImprovementMethods/Measures/

Krenzischek, D. A., & Newhouse, R. (2005). Dissemination of findings. In R. Newhouse & S. Poe (Eds.), *Measuring patient safety* (pp. 67-78). Boston: Jones & Bartlett.

McGlynn, E. A. (1998). Choosing and evaluating clinical performance measures. *Joint Commission Journal of Quality Improvement, 24*, 470-479.

National Bioethics Commission. (2001). *Ethical and policy issues in research involving human participants*. Bethesda, MD: National Bioethics Advisory Commission.

Newhouse, R. P. (2007a). Creating infrastructure supportive of evidence-based nursing practice: Leadership strategies. *Worldviews on Evidence-Based Nursing, 4*(1), 21-29.

Newhouse, R. P. (2007b). Diffusing confusion among evidence-based practice, quality improvement and research. *Journal of Nursing Administration, 37*(10), 432-435.

Newhouse, R.P., Pettit, J.C., Rocco, L., & Poe, S. (2006). The slippery slope: Differentiating between quality improvement and research. *Journal of Nursing Administration, 36*(4), 211-219.

Pronovost, P. J., Miller, M. R., Dorman, T., Berenholtz, S. M., & Rubin, H. (2001). Developing and implementing measures of quality of care in the intensive care unit. *Current Opinions in Critical Care, 7*, 297-303.

Rogers, E. M. (1983). *Diffusions of innovations* (3rd ed.). New York: The Free Press.

Stetler, C. B. (2001). Updating the Stetler Model of research utilization to facilitate evidence-based practice. *Nursing Outlook, 49*, 272-279.

Other Resources

Deming, W. E. (2000). *The new economics for industry, government, education* (2nd ed.). Cambridge, MA: The MIT Press.

Langley, G. J., Nolan, K. M., Nolan, T. W., Norman, C. L., & Provost, L. P. (1996). *The improvement guide: A practical approach to enhancing organizational performance*. San Francisco, CA: Jossey-Bass.

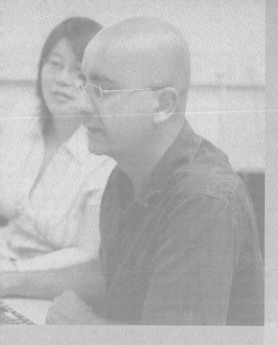

IV

Infrastructure

Chapter 9

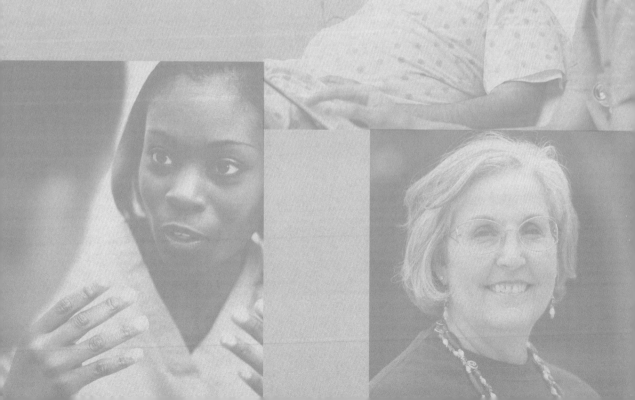

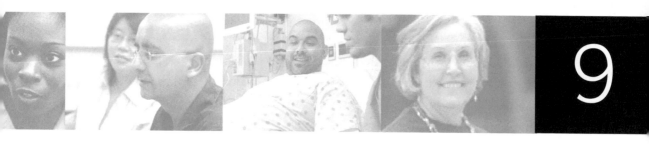

Creating a Supportive
EBP Environment

The dynamic and competitive health-care environment requires health-care practitioners who are accountable and provide efficient and effective care. The environment mandates improvement in care processes and outcomes. Why be concerned about evidence-based practice?

The most obvious answer is that new evidence is continually surfacing in our nursing and medical environments. There has been a tremendous increase in the generation of new knowledge that practitioners need to incorporate in their daily routine for their practice to be evidence-based. Yet, there is a well-documented, long delay in implementing new knowledge into practice environments. The Agency for Healthcare Research and Quality (Clancy & Cronin, 2005) cited that the average time from generation of new evidence to implementation of that evidence into practice is 17 years. Additionally, the *British Medical Journal* (Davidoff, Haynes, Sackett, & Smith, 1995) reported that to keep up with the journals relevant to practice, each practitioner would need to read 17 articles per day, 365 days per year. That was more than

10 years ago; today, there are even more health-care journals for practitioners to read. Health care is provided within the structure of a system or organization, and the health-care organization can either facilitate or inhibit the uptake of evidence. EBP requires the creation of an environment that fosters lifelong learning to increase the use of evidence in our practice.

Many health-care organizations, because of the emphasis on quality and safety, have created strategic initiatives for EBP. Current national pay for performance initiatives, both voluntary and mandatory, provide reimbursement to hospitals and practitioners for implementing health-care practices that are supported by evidence. Consumer pressure and increased patient expectations lend an even greater emphasis on this need for true evidence-based practice. However, McGlynn et al. (2003), in an often-cited study, reported that Americans receive only about 50% of recommended health care. Therefore, even with an increased emphasis on EBP in health care, the majority of hospitals and practitioners are not implementing the current available evidence and guidelines for care in their practices. This suggests an even greater imperative for building infrastructure that supports EBP and infuses it into practice environments.

The American Nurses Association significantly revised the Scope and Standards for Nursing Practice in 2004, making substantive changes to references to the imperative for evidence in nursing practice. The revised standards created a significantly stronger role for nurses to create the environment and advocate for resources to support research (American Nurses Association, 2004). The document also changes the words *knowledge-driven nursing practice* to "research that promotes evidence-based, clinically effective and efficient, nurse-sensitive patient/client/resident outcomes and other healthcare outcomes" and requires nurses to facilitate dissemination and integration of evidence-based practices.

A new type of health-care worker exists today—one educated to think critically and not accept the status quo. Generation X nurses are questioning current nursing practices—and "We've always done it that way" is not a good enough answer. They want evidence that what they are doing in the workplace is efficient, effective, and efficacious. These nurses will push the profession away from doing things unsupported by evidence because of tradition and past practices. This push should be to require that evidence support all clinical, educational, and administrative decision making.

There is a compelling need for EBP in our health-care environments. However, any kind of organizational change requires proper planning, development, and commitment. The creation of a standardized framework for EBP inquiry in the organization is critical to implement best practices (both clinically and administratively), identify and improve cost components of care, foster outcomes improvement, and ensure the success of the EBP initiative.

The environmental variable is extremely important to developing an evidence-based practice. It demands the support and commitment of leadership, the identification and reduction of barriers to implementation, and the development and mentoring of staff. This chapter

- explores how to create and facilitate a supportive EBP environment

- discusses lessons learned for leadership in EBP

- describes how to overcome common barriers to implementation

- identifies specific strategies to support and mentor staff in developing EBP

Leadership

A supportive and committed leadership, including the top administration and the chief nurse executive (CNE), must be involved in the creation and development of an evidence-based practice environment. Leadership for the successful infusion of evidence-based practice throughout the organization must focus on three key strategies: *establish the culture*, *develop the capacity*, and *sustain the change*.

Establish the Culture

Key assumptions of evidence-based nursing practice include:

1. Nursing is both a science and an applied profession.

2. Knowledge is important to professional practice, and there are limits to knowledge that must be identified.

3. Not all evidence is created equal, and there is a need to use the best available evidence.

4. Evidence-based practice contributes to improved outcomes (Newhouse, 2007).

Establishing a culture of evidence-based practice requires that the leadership of the organization participate in the development of a *mission*. The mission of an organization must include several key points. First, the mission should speak to the spirit of inquiry of the staff and the lifelong learning necessary for an evidence-based practice. Second, the mission should address a work environment that demands and supports nurses' accountability for practice and decision making. Finally, the mission needs to include the goal of improving patient care outcomes through evidence-based clinical and administrative decision making. See Table 9.1 for an example of the mission statement for The Johns Hopkins Hospital Department of Nursing and Patient Care Services.

Some indicators of an environment supportive of nursing inquiry include

- The staff has access to nursing reference books and the Internet on the patient care unit.

- Journals are available in hard copy or online.

- There is a medical/nursing library available.

- Knowledgeable library personnel are available to support staff and assist with evidence searches.

- Other resources are available for inquiry and EBP.

Estabrooks (1998) surveyed staff nurses about their use of various sources of knowledge. She found that the sources used most often by nurses were experience, other workplace sources, physician sources, intuition, and what has worked for years. Nurses ranked literature, texts, or journals, in the bottom five of all sources accessed for information. Pravikoff, Tanner, and Pierce (2005) studied EBP readiness among nurses and found that 61% of nurses needed to look up clinical information at least one time per week. However, 67% of the nurses always or frequently sought information from a colleague instead of reference text, and 83% rarely or never sought a librarian's assistance. An organization that provides resources for practice inquiry can highlight the resources, and those that do not must address this critical need.

Table 9.1.   Mission Statement for The Johns Hopkins Hospital Department of Nursing and Patient Care Services

Mission: To ensure the delivery of optimal patient care and excellent patient care services.

Mission is fulfilled through:

- Coordination of Nursing and other patient care services (Social Work, Patient & Visitor Services)

- Maintenance of quality assurance standards

- Appropriate allocation and management of nursing resources

- Development and maintenance of a governance structure with operating procedures and staffing to meet the needs of the organization and the Department of Nursing

- Collaboration with the Directors of Nursing to develop, implement, and evaluate the Department of Nursing's strategic and operational plans

- Collaboration with the Directors of Nursing to establish standards of nursing care and practice and to assure that these standards guide the provision of nursing care

- Provision of central nursing support for functional units in areas of organizational development, management systems, human resource management, staff development, education, and research

- Collaboration with the Dean of The Johns Hopkins University School of Nursing to provide an organizational structure that advances professional nursing practice, education, and research

- Compliance with regulatory requirements of Federal, State, and accrediting entities; maintenance of current accreditations and licenses, e.g. Joint Commission on Accreditation of Healthcare Organizations (JCAHO) accreditation; State of Maryland licensure

To operationalize a mission statement, an organization's leadership must develop a strategic plan for the implementation of EBP. This plan needs to identify specific goals and objectives, time frames, responsibilities, and a process for evaluation. The plan also requires the commitment of the organization's administration for allocation of adequate resources to the EBP initiative, including people, time, money, education, and mentoring. As a strategic goal, evidence-based practice should be implemented at all levels of the organization.

The support and visibility of the CNE in establishing the culture of EBP is paramount. The staff must see the CNE as a champion and leader with a goal of infusing, building, and sustaining an evidence-based practice environment. Therefore, the CNE should participate in EBP education and training. For example, if the plan is to offer education to the management group about EBP, the CNE should attend the education and begin the day by discussing the leadership's vision of EBP. The CNE's presence demonstrates the leadership's commitment to EBP and the value of EBP to the organization. Participating gives the CNE an appreciation for the process, including the time and resource commitment necessary for the organization to move toward an evidence-based practice.

The organization's leadership can further role model support for EBP efforts by ensuring that all administrative decision making is evidence-based. For example, if the organization's leadership asks middle management for evidence (both organizational data and the best available research and non-research evidence) to support important decisions in its areas of responsibility, it is more likely that staff nurses at all levels will also question and require evidence for their practice decisions. Additionally, all organizational and department of nursing policies and procedures need to be evidence-based, having the source citations on the policy or procedure available if there is a need to retrieve the reference. These policies and procedures should be reviewed in staff meetings as a standing agenda item, with identification of the evidence citation in the policy. Within these small leadership examples and activities, verbal and non-verbal EBP language assimilates into everyday activities and establishes an evidence-based culture.

Finally, the leadership needs to be involved throughout the development and implementation of the EBP strategic plan. As the initiative rolls out, it is important for leaders to check the pulse of the organization and be prepared to modify the strategy as necessary. To enable the process, it is critical that the leadership identify potential barriers to implementation, have a plan to reduce or remove them, and support the project directors and change champions in every way possible.

Develop the Capacity

To move the evidence-based practice initiative forward, the organization's leadership must develop the capacity and ensure that the appropriate infrastructure is available and supported within the organization. Capacity building includes the careful implementation of the previously developed strategic plan. The organizational capacity consists of human and material resources as well as the establishment of a ready culture.

To develop capacity, the nursing leadership team must carefully evaluate and adopt an EBP model or framework. EBP model selection should consider

- the fit and feasibility of the model with the vision, mission, and values of the organization

- the educational background, leadership, experience, and practice needs of the nursing staff

- the presence of any partnerships or collaboration for the EBP initiative, such as a school of nursing or physician interest

- the culture and environment of the organization

- the accessibility and availability of credible sources of knowledge

Leadership must identify and select change champions with care to develop capacity. Attention must be given to select champions from across the organization— different professionals, levels, and specialties. Consider who within the organization has the knowledge and skills to move an EBP initiative forward, who will be the best supporters, and who has the most at stake to see that EBP is successful.

The identification of champions can occur at two levels. The first set of champions needs to be at the departmental level. The Johns Hopkins Hospital nursing leadership has successfully used the departmental nursing committee structure to develop these champions. The second group of champions is at the unit level. These people will most likely be unit-based expert clinicians and unit leaders. They must be individuals the staff sees as role models of professional practice and accountability. They are the nurses who are committed to clinical inquiry and many times are initially identified because they are interested in the priority topic or issue. It is also important that these individuals be collaborators and team players, because EBP work involves other professional colleagues.

The implementation of the EBP strategic initiative needs to address the skill and knowledge building of champions, mentors, and staff and must consider how to construct an EBP infrastructure. For example, how will the champions, mentors, and staff be trained? Who will provide the initial training? Moreover, how and by whom will they be supported after their training is complete? It is also important that the development or acquisition of tools to support the EBP initiative be discussed. For example, what kind of tools will be needed for evidence appraisal, and what summary and reporting documents will be necessary? Make sure that these tools are understandable, easy to use, and facilitate the EBP work. Specific tools that guide the EBP process have been an important key to the success and implementation of the Johns Hopkins Nursing EBP Model and Guidelines for staff nurses. The JHNEBP tools (Appendixes A–I) serve as guides and reminders for the staff of what they need to consider as they embark on EBP projects. The more organized and systematic the process and the accompanying tools, the less there is to worry about that part of the EBP initiative.

When considering how to build capacity, leadership should develop job descriptions, orientation programs and materials, and performance evaluation tools that incorporate EBP. These personnel tools should be developed or revised to emphasize the staff's responsibility and accountability for administrative and practice decision making to improve patient care outcomes and processes. The tools must be consistent across the employment continuum. For example, the job description should state what is expected of the nurse in terms of standards and measurement of competence; the orientation should introduce the nurse to the organization and how standards are upheld and competencies are developed at the organization; and the performance evaluation tool should measure the nurse's level of performance on the standards with specific measures of competence. Table 9.2 provides examples of standards of performance and competence from The Johns Hopkins Hospital Department of Nursing job descriptions.

Table 9.2. Excerpts from JHH Job Descriptions for Staff Nurses

Nurse Clinician I

I. Clinical Practice

F. Applies a scientific basis/EBP approach towards nursing practice.

1. Complies with changes in clinical practice and standards.
2. Participates in data collection when the opportunity is presented.
3. Poses relevant clinical questions when evidence and practice differ.
4. Consults appropriate experts when the basis for practice is questioned.
5. Uses appropriate resources to answer evidence-based practice questions.
6. Additional requirement for IM: Reviews current evidence relevant to practice.

Nurse Clinician II

I. Clinical Practice

F. Applies a scientific basis/EBP approach towards nursing practice.

1. Seeks and/or articulates rationale and scientific basis for clinical practice or changes in standards.
2. Supports research-based clinical practice (teaches, role models, applies to own practices).
3. Participates in data collection, when the opportunity is presented.
4. Identifies difference in practice and best evidence.
5. Generates clinical questions, searches evidence, and reviews evidence related to area of practice.
6. Consults appropriate experts to answer evidence-based practice questions.
7. Articulates evidence-based rationale for care.

Table 9.2. Excerpts from JHH Job Descriptions for Staff Nurses (continued)

Nurse Clinician III

I. Clinical Practice

F. Interprets research and uses scientific inquiry to validate and/or change clinical practice.

  1. Evaluates research findings with potential implications for changing clinical practice, compares practice to findings, and takes appropriate action.

  2. Designs tool and/or participates in data collection and other specific assignments (e.g., literature review) in the conduct of research when the opportunity presents.

  3. Mentors staff to identify differences in practice and best evidence, generates clinical questions, searches evidence, reviews and critiques evidence related to area of clinical, administrative, or education practice.

  4. Serves as a resource and mentor in evidence-based discussions articulating rationale for practice.

  5. Participates in implementing evidence-based practice through role modeling and support of practice changes.

  6. Incorporates EBP into daily patient care and leadership responsibilities.

  7. Participates in/supports evidence-based practice projects within unit/department.

III. Resources

B. Uses critical thinking and scientific inquiry to systematically and continually improve care and business processes and to achieve desired financial outcomes.

Sustain the Change

After an EBP initiative starts, the organization's leadership must commit to support and sustain this change in how the organization approaches its work. The leaders, along with the change champions and those responsible for the initiative, must listen to staff and be responsive to comments, questions, and complaints. For EBP to become a part of the entire organization, ownership must be developed at all levels, and staff must see this as a partnership. The perception that changing practice will improve quality of care and make a difference in patients' lives can be felt by all staff, and the passion will be palpable to all when EBP becomes a part of the daily routine.

As resources are allocated to an EBP initiative, questions may arise about the expenditures and the need for EBP in light of cost. To sustain the work and value to the organization, linking EBP project work to organizational priorities is important. As discussed earlier, it is helpful to identify EBP projects that improve safety or risk management problems; address wide variations in practice or clinical practice that are different from the community standard; and solve high-risk, high-volume, or high-cost problems. Ask whether there is any evidence to support the organization's current practice. Are these the best achievable outcomes, and is there a way to be more efficient or cost-effective? Improvements or benefits to the organization in any of these important areas could result if best practices were identified that would improve outcomes of care or decrease costs or risks associated with the problem. Another way of showing the cost-effectiveness of EBP work is to improve patient and/or staff satisfaction or health-related quality of life because of an EBP project.

Sustaining the change also involves development of an evaluation plan. The plan needs to include performance measures, both process and outcomes measures, that monitor and evaluate the implementation, commitment, and results. The measures should aim to determine the usefulness, satisfaction, and success of the EBP environment. Are the initiatives changing or supporting current practice? What best practices or exemplars have resulted? Has the organization saved money or become more efficient, and where is the performance data to show that this is making a difference to the organization? The evaluation plan should include a time line and triggers that would signal that a modification of the plan is necessary.

The development of a communication plan should be a part of the planning process and maintenance of the change. The plan should address the following:

- goals of the communication

- target audiences

- available communication mediums

- preferred frequency of communication

- important messages

Minimally, the goals for an EBP communication plan are to increase staff awareness of the initiative, educate the staff regarding its contribution to the initiative, and inform the staff of successes and celebrate them. Consider the development of EBP "messages." Messages can help to target the communication, link the initiative to the organization's mission, and give a consistent vision while providing new and varied information about the initiative. Table 9.3 includes examples of messages from The Johns Hopkins Hospital Department of Nursing Web site, http://www.hopkinsnursing.org/.

Table 9.3.   Examples of Communication Messages

INTERNAL MESSAGE: Unit-Based Committees

Unit-based nursing committees not only form the basis for shared governance here, they help you take the lead on such issues as peer review, patient safety, education, performance improvement, evidence-based practice, and more. All over this complex medical center, nurses are creating innovative techniques that can ease patients' stays in the hospital and improve the quality of their lives. Your ideas matter—and we are listening.

EXTERNAL MESSAGE: We Are Magnetic

In 2003, Johns Hopkins became the first and only health care organization in Maryland to achieve the Magnet Recognition Program designation for excellence in nursing practice.

From our beginnings more than 125 years ago, Hopkins nurses have stood in the forefront of the profession. Our first superintendent of nurses, Isabel Hampton, helped launch the American Nurses Association, and then served as its first president. Adelaide Nutting, her successor, helped create the American Journal of Nursing. We like to think that these visionaries, who worked so tirelessly to set national standards and elevate nursing's status, would be as proud as we are of our Magnet designation.

The highest honor bestowed by the American Nurses Credentialing Center, Magnet status affirms the depth and breadth of Hopkins Nursing—our evidence-based practice, our interdisciplinary collaboration and participatory decision-making, and our spirit of innovation and excellence.

Part of the communication plan is keeping the staff regularly informed and up-to-date about EBP activities throughout the organization. Investigating ways to involve the staff through the communication plan, such as asking staff opinions of potential or completed work through an online survey, can allow the leadership to maintain a finger on the pulse of the initiative.

A final recommendation is to consider developing an EBP Web site within the organization's intranet. The Web site can be an excellent internal vehicle for communicating EBP information, including questions under consideration, projects in progress, projects completed and their outcomes, and available EBP educational opportunities that are available. The Web site can also serve as a snapshot and history of an organization's EBP activities—for example, seeking or maintaining Magnet designation.

After the movement toward a supportive EBP environment begins, the biggest challenge is to keep the momentum going. The leadership must consider how to reward the EBP champions and mentors and incentivize the staff for developing a practice that incorporates the best available evidence. Consider whether the organization's system includes incentives or disincentives and whether an accountability-based environment exists. These are crucial discussion points during the planning, implementation, and maintenance of the change. To sustain the change, the staff must own the change and work to sustain the change to a practice environment that values critical thinking and uses evidence for all administrative and clinical decision making.

Overcoming Barriers

One of the ongoing responsibilities of the leadership is to identify and develop a plan to overcome barriers to the implementation and maintenance of an EBP environment within the organization. This responsibility cannot be taken lightly and must be a part of the implementation plan.

The greatest barrier identified by those involved in EBP is *time*. Time constraints are repeatedly cited as the barrier that prevents implementation of EBP and prevents continued use of an investigative model for practice. The provision of clinical release time to staff participating in an EBP project is essential. Experience shows that staff nurses need time to think about and discuss the EBP project. They also need time to read the latest evidence and appraise the validity, strength, and quality of the evidence. Nurses need uninterrupted time away from the clinical unit. This work cannot be done in stolen moments away from the patients, in 15-minute intervals. Reading research and critiquing evidence is challenging and demanding work for most nurses, and requires that blocks of time be set aside for staff to do effective work.

Discussed previously was the need for leadership. A *lack of supportive leadership* for EBP within an organization is a major barrier to the creation and maintenance of an EBP environment. Leadership can be facilitated through the vision, mission, and strategic plan. The top leaders must incorporate EBP into their roles and normative behavior. To create a culture of organizational support for EBP, the day-to-day language must be consistent with using evidence and be a part of the organizational values. That is, *talk the talk*—make the point to ask, where is the evidence? Leaders must also *walk* the talk, demonstrating this on a daily basis in their actions and behaviors. Does the organization value science and research and hold its staff accountable for use of best evidence in practice and clinical decision making? As routine decisions are made, do leaders question whether the decision is being made using the best possible data/evidence or on experience or history, financial restrictions, or even emotion? Do leaders use the best evidence available to them for administrative decision making? This can easily be seen if one looks at the titles for administrative staff within the organization. Is there a director or department for research or quality improvement? If there is, where are these individuals on the organizational chart? Whom do they report to? Are these roles centralized or decentralized in the organizational structure?

A *lack of organizational infrastructure* to support EBP is another important barrier to deal with. Resources, in terms of people, money, and time, need to be negotiated and allocated to support the initiative. Access to library resources or computers for online database resources must be planned for. How will staff get access to the current evidence? Experts, the champions and mentors, are also a part of the infrastructure that must be present.

Nurses themselves can be a significant barrier to implementing EBP. Nurses often lack the skills, knowledge, and confidence to read the results of research studies and translate them into practice. It is also common that some nurses resist EBP through negative attitudes and skepticism toward research. In some organizations, nurses may feel they have limited authority to make or change practice decisions and are skeptical that anything can result from the pursuit of evidence.

Barriers that come from nurses are best dealt with through prevention and planning to assess and identify staff needs, and through support and mentoring by experts and champions throughout and after the EBP process to incorporate the change into their practice. Another potential barrier is the relationships of staff nurses with other nurses in the organizational hierarchy, such as clinical nurse specialists, and with physicians and other professional staff. Professionals need to value the contributions of others to patient care and clinical decision making. If the input of all staff is not valued, especially the input of nurses, there will be a lack of interest in and lack of confidence to participate in an EBP initiative.

Lack of communication is a common barrier to implementation of any change but is particularly important to EBP initiatives. This can be prevented by using the strategies discussed above in the design of a communication plan for an EBP initiative. As the staff develops EBP and approaches the clinical environment with critical thinking, they want to know that what they are doing is valued. The staff values responsiveness and listening on the part of the leadership to concerns or questions as the change is implemented. Staff members take ownership of the change if they sense that the leadership listens to them and answers or modifies as necessary.

A final barrier is *lack of incentives,* or rewards, in the organization for support of an EBP environment. Criticism and discussion arise over this barrier by those who think that staff should not have to be rewarded for doing its job. However, establishing an EBP environment and continuing EBP project work are challenging and require a level of commitment on the part of all involved. Incentives can be dealt with in several areas already discussed: communication, education and mentoring, job descriptions and evaluation tools, and so on. However, the leadership team should understand the need for staff incentives and plan for recognition and rewards that are a part of the EBP implementation process.

Strategies for Developing and Mentoring Staff

Begin the development and mentoring of staff with a careful selection of expert clinicians, leaders, role models, and those who are committed to inquiry. Those selected will become the change champions and mentors for other staff. The ability to have team members focus and collaborate is important, because many practice changes involve more than just nursing and include physicians, other allied health professionals, administrators, and policy makers. As the activities to build an EBP environment increase, it is important to begin identifying additional staff to include in EBP education and mentoring. The key to success at this stage is to increase buy-in by involving as many potential champions as possible in an EBP process focused on a problem that is of importance to them. These factors were all present in the first JHNEBP project conducted at The Johns Hopkins Hospital.

After the JHNEBP Model was developed and ready for testing, the first group to receive education and training on the model was the PACU staff (Exemplar 5). They were chosen for three reasons. First, the PACU had a nurse manager committed to EBP; second, the PACU had well-established professional practice and expectations of staff nurse involvement in unit activities; and finally, PACU nurses had 2 hours of protected time on their schedule each week that could be used for the training. The PACU staff proposed to examine an administrative and clinical question that was a cost, volume, and satisfaction issue. The issue also became a priority because it affected throughput and thus received complete support to study for the first EBP initiative. The question generated by the staff was, "Should ambulatory adults void before discharge from the PACU?" The PACU staff was given education in short weekly or biweekly sessions. Table 9.4 shows a sample agenda for "Fast Track" EBP Educational Sessions. Each week, the PACU staff was asked to evaluate the education, the model, and their satisfaction with the process. They were asked the following questions:

- Is the model clear, usable, adequate, and feasible?

- Is the staff satisfied with the evidence-based process?

- Is the staff satisfied with the outcome of the process?

Table 9.4. Sample Agenda for "Fast Track" EBP Educational Sessions

Topic and Time Suggestion	Objectives
Session #1 Introduction to EBP 30 Min.	Define EBP & describe the importance of EBP
Session #2 EBP Model 30 Min.	Discuss the Johns Hopkins Nursing EBP Model and Guidelines (PET Process)
Session #3 Searching the Evidence 20 minutes	Identify and describe different types of evidence and how to locate
Session #4 EBP Process 20 Min.	Discuss the PET process in detail
Session #5 Evidence Appraisal Tools 20 Min.	Describe how to use the EBP tools
Session #6 Appraising the Evidence 45 Min.	Describe how to evaluate different types of evidence
Session #7 Evaluation and Next Steps 30 Min.	Review of expectations for the project, "getting started," and translating evidence into practice

The results of the evaluation of the model and process demonstrated significant differences across time in the nurses' perceptions of the adequacy of the EBP resources, the feasibility of the process, and their satisfaction with the process and outcome. Figure 9.1 shows the mean changes in evaluation responses across time. After the initial training, the nurses began the process with positive perceptions, which dropped significantly in all areas when they began to use the model to search and evaluate the evidence independently. At the end of five sessions, the nurses' perceptions of the adequacy of EBP resources, the feasibility of the process, and their satisfaction with the process and outcome returned to higher levels than their initial ratings. These results support the need for mentorship during the EBP process as nurses learn new skills, including the research and evidence appraisal work (Newhouse et al., 2005). At the end of the pilot, the EBP leadership team concluded that staff nurses can effectively use the JHNEBP Model with the help of knowledgeable mentors, and that implementation of a practical EBP model is necessary to translate research into practice. The evaluation also included qualitative responses that showed enthusiasm for the EBP process and a renewed sense of professionalism and accomplishment among the nurses, and included a few suggestions for minor revisions to the process.

Nurse Evaluation of EBP Model Over Pilot

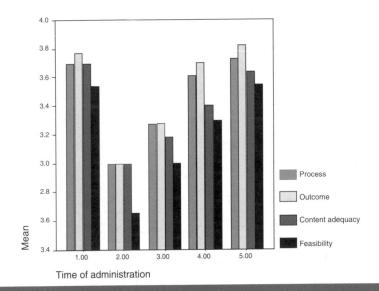

Figure 9.1.   Nurse Evaluation of Implementation of the EBP Model during the Pilot

Following the successful pilot evaluation of the JHNEBP, The Johns Hopkins Hospital Department of Nursing identified the development of EBP as a strategic initiative. It was decided that an educational plan targeting staff to become EBP change champions would begin with the department of nursing committee structure, including the Nursing Research Committee, Nursing Practice Committee, Nursing Standards of Care Committee (SOC), Performance Improvement Committee (PI), and Education Committee. Each of these committees has a different but important role for implementing EBP throughout the organization. The EBP leadership team put together three train-the-trainer workshops for the department of nursing committee members. The 2-day educational workshops focused on the practical development and use of EBP concepts, including the ability to search for and appraise evidence, summarize the evidence, and plan for translation of findings into practice. Table 9.5 details a sample agenda for a 2-day EBP workshop.

Table 9.5. Sample Agenda for 2-Day EBP Workshop

Day 1	Topic
8:00 am – 8:15 am	Opening Remarks – Overview of Day
8:15 am – 9:00 am	Intro to Evidence-Based Practice (EBP)
9:00 am – 9:45 am	JH Nursing EBP Model and Process
9:45 am – 10:00 am	Break
10:00 am – 11:30 am	Appraising the Evidence
11:30 am – 12:30 pm	Lunch
12:30 pm – 1:45 pm	Computer/Library Lab (Distribute article packets)
1:45 pm – 2:00 pm	Break
2:00 pm – 2:30 pm	Computer/Library Lab – Searching your own problem
2:30 pm – 2:45 pm	Q and A
	Review of assignment and format for Day 2

Day 1 ends early to allow time for participants to read their assigned articles

Day 2	Topic
8:00 am – 8:15 am	Opening Remarks – Overview of Day
8:15 am – 9:15 am	How to Run an Effective EBP Meeting/ Moving an Agenda
9:15 am – 10:15 am	Mock Evidence Appraisal Group Meeting
10:15 am – 10:30 am	Break
10:30 am – 11:30 am	Mock Evidence Appraisal Group Meeting
11:30 am – 12:30 pm	Lunch
12:30 pm – 2:00 pm	Should Practice Change, Based on Evidence?
2:00 pm – 2:15 pm	Break
2:15 pm – 3:15 pm	Creating a Supportive EBP Environment
3:15 pm – 3:45 pm	Program Wrap-Up and Evaluation (Day 2)

Each of the nursing committees was asked to develop an EBP question of importance to their committee work and goals for the year. The SOC and Research Committee asked, "What are the best practices related to effective pain management for patients with a history of substance abuse?" The SOC Committee questioned, "Should cooling blankets be used to reduce fever? If so, what is the best type of cooling blanket? And, how often should vital signs be taken?" The PI and Education Committee examined, "What strategies should be used in the OR to decrease the incidence of pressure ulcer development postoperatively?" In each of these examples, the EBP question was generated by the committee because of different needs for evidence to inform the practice. Problem origins included QI data that suggested a problem, a perceived variation from community standard, and the need to identify best practices to improve efficiency and effectiveness of care. Again, the participants evaluated the use of the model and satisfaction with the process and outcomes.

The important role that the mentor plays in facilitating these projects and the translation of the evidence into practice became clearer with each project. The nursing literature supports the conclusions of this EBP leadership team that mentoring and support are needed throughout an EBP process to help nurses to be successful and to promote excellence (Block, Claffrey, Korow, & McCaffrey, 2005; Carroll, 2004; Owens & Patton, 2003).

The initial educational training was targeted for nurses that served on the governance committees. Because of the significant role of nurse managers in generating questions, working with staff to schedule time to dedicate to the EBP projects, and assuring that recommendations were supported and implemented, a manager-focused educational session was conducted. The nurse managers needed EBP training to enable them to understand and support their staff in EBP initiatives, as well as use the EBP processes in their own decision-making. A group of nurse managers completed the training and asked, "Do artificial nails worn by health-care providers increase the risk of nosocomial infections?"

In addition to initial strategies focused on leaders and change champions, a competitive Fellowship in EBP was developed for staff nurses. Two fellowships were budgeted each year as a funded part-time opportunity for a Johns Hopkins

Hospital RN. The selected candidate would work with a mentor to develop EBP skills and complete a proposed project that answers a specific EBP question. The first fellow developed a project focused on an ICU practice problem: For patients in the ICU, what nursing assessment parameters identify patients with new onset delirium? The second fellow focused on a question generated by the SOC committee: Should enzymatic cleaner be used for ophthalmology instruments? Fellowships provide staff nurses with 50% salary support over 3 months, during which they are released from clinical assignments to work on the EBP project. They use the JHNEBP Model and guidelines to translate their recommendations to practice and evaluation. The first two fellows advanced professionally, with one returning to graduate school and the second being promoted to nurse manager.

The need to prepare nurses with EBP knowledge and skills is recognized at The Johns Hopkins University School of Nursing (JHUSON). The JHUSON also adopted the JHNEBP Model and guidelines. The baccalaureate program integrated the model and PET process into didactic and clinical courses. One example is the baccalaureate research class where real-life EBP questions are generated from JHH units and given to the research instructor. As a course assignment, nursing students search and critique the available evidence from PubMed and CINAHL and provide a report summarizing the literature to the JHH functional unit for implementation of the project. The master's program underwent a curriculum revision, and the research course was revised and renamed *Applications of Research to Practice*. The PhD and new Doctor of Nursing (DNP) programs also incorporate evidence-based practice in their curriculums. The PhD program has an elective called Evidence-Based Nursing. The DNP program focuses the curriculum on EBP and has two core courses that emphasize the content. Additionally, the DNP students complete systematic reviews of the literature in the focus area of their capstone projects.

To more effectively integrate evidence-based practice concepts into the curriculum, a faculty development workshop was held at the JHUSON. The faculty fast-tracked through the concepts but actually participated in an EBP project to experience the JHNEBP Model and guidelines and the tools available for them to use with their students.

The EBP leadership team continues to develop and mentor staff. Most of the education provided to the staff is now a 1-day workshop. The morning session covers EBP concepts and the JHNEBP Model and guidelines, and reviews evidence searching and appraisal techniques. In the afternoon, attendees critique and appraise the evidence for an EBP question and decide as a group whether a practice change is warranted, based on the evidence available to them. Table 9.6 is a sample agenda for a 1-day (8-hour) EBP workshop. One-day workshops have successfully been implemented in many settings outside of Johns Hopkins and Baltimore, including rural hospitals, community hospitals, non-teaching hospitals, and other large academic medical centers.

Table 9.6.   Sample Agenda for 1-Day (8-hr) EBP Workshop

8:00 am	**Continental Breakfast**
8:20 am – 8:30 am	**Welcome/Opening Remarks – Chief Nurse Executive**
8:30 am – 9:00 am	**Introduction to Evidence-Based Practice**
	■ Design and purpose of the workshop
	■ Definition of EBP
	■ Discuss importance of EBP
9:00 am – 9:45 am	**Guidelines for Implementation**
	■ Describe model
	■ Discuss plans for using the model
	■ Describe the steps in the process
	■ Discuss how to develop an answerable question
9:45 am – 10:00 am	**Break**
10:00 am – 11:00 am	**Appraising Evidence**
	■ Describe the different types of evidence
	■ Determine where to look for evidence
11:00 am – 11:30 am	**Searching for Evidence**
	■ Discuss library services
	■ How to have a search run by the library
	■ How to order articles
	■ Other services
	■ Demonstrate how to do basic literature search

11:30am – 12:15 pm	**Lunch**
12:15 pm – 2:45 pm	**Appraising the Evidence**
	■ Brief explanation of the forms used
	■ Appraisal/evaluation of assigned articles
	■ Completion of individual and overall evidence summary forms
2:45 pm – 3:00 pm	**Break**
3:00 pm – 3:30 pm	**Summarizing the Evidence and Beyond**
	■ Determine if practice changes are indicated
	■ Determine how changes could be implemented
	■ Discuss how changes can be evaluated
3:30 pm – 4:00 pm	**Translation Strategies and Wrap-Up**
	Identify barriers and facilitators to implementation of an EBP project and strategies for success
4:00 p.m.	**Program Evaluation**

Summary

There have been many lessons learned in the development of the JHNEBP Model and guidelines. The need to create a supportive EBP environment is one of the most important. Essential to that effort is a supportive leadership that establishes a culture of EBP; develops the capacity to implement EBP, including the expansion of infrastructure and allocation of resources such as time, money, and people; and is able to sustain the change and overcome barriers and resistance to the change. The keys to the successful implementation of EBP and to overcoming the many barriers and resistance to EBP are leadership and planning.

With the goals of ensuring the highest quality of care and using evidence to promote optimal outcomes, reduce inappropriate variation in care, and promote patient and staff satisfaction, a culture of critical thinking and ongoing learning creates an environment where evidence supports clinical and administrative decisions. Working in an EBP environment changes the way nurses think about and approach that work. Leadership sets the priority, facilitates the process, and sets expectations. After the nursing staffs develop expertise in the EBP process, their professional growth and engagement begins a personal and organizational trajectory leading to evidence-based decisions, a higher level of critical review of evidence, and engagement of nursing in the interdisciplinary team as a valued contributor.

References

American Nurses Association. (2004). *Scope and standards of nursing practice.* Washington, DC: American Nurses Publishing.

Block, L., Claffey, C., Korow, M., & McCaffrey, R. (2005). The value of mentorship within nursing organizations. *Nursing Forum, 40*(4), 134-140.

Carroll, K. (2004). Mentoring: A human becoming perspective. *Nursing Science Quarterly, 17*(4), 318-322.

Clancy, C., & Cronin, K. (2005). Evidence-based decision making: Global evidence, local decisions. *Health Affairs, 24*(1), 151-162.

Davidoff, F., Haynes, B., Sackett, D., & Smith, R. (1995). Evidence based medicine: A new journal to help doctors identify the information they need. *British Medical Journal, 310*(6987), 1085-1086.

Estabrooks, C. (1998). Will evidence-based nursing practice make practice perfect? *Canadian Journal of Nursing Research, 30,* 15-36.

The Johns Hopkins Hospital. (n.d.). *Johns Hopkins Nursing.* Retrieved October 21, 2007, from http://www.hopkinsnursing.org/

McGlynn, E., Asch, S., Adams, J., Keesey, J., Hicks, J., Decristofaro, A., & Kerr, E. (2003). The quality of health care delivered to adults in the United States. *New England Journal of Medicine, 348*(26), 2635-2645.

Newhouse, R. P. (2007). Creating infrastructure supportive of evidence-based nursing practice: Leadership strategies. *Worldviews on Evidence-Based Nursing, 4*(1), 21-29.

Newhouse, R., Poe, S., Dearholt, S., Pugh, L., & White. K. (2005). Evidence-based practice: A practical approach to implementation. *Journal of Nursing Administration, 35*(1), 35-40.

Owens, J., & Patton, J. (2003). Take a chance on nursing mentorships. *Nursing Education Perspectives, 24*(4), 198-204.

Pravikoff, D., Tanner, A., & Pierce, S. (2005). Readiness of US nurses for evidence-based practice. *American Journal of Nursing, 105*(9), 40-51.

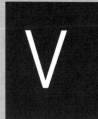

V

Exemplars

Chapter 10

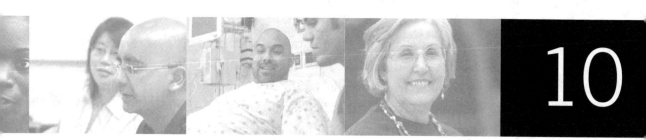

Exemplars

To Void or Not to Void?

Dina A. Krenzischek, MAS, RN, CPAN
Mary Ares, MSN, RN
Robin Lewis, BSN, RN
Felisa Tanseco, BSN, RN, CPAN
Robin Newhouse, PhD, RN

Practice Question

Patients are routinely required to void prior to discharge regardless of type of surgery, anesthetic technique, or associated risk factors. This results in holding patients unnecessarily in the Post Anesthesia Care Unit (PACU), increasing their length of stay, delaying their return to the comfort of their home and family, increasing costs, and possibly impeding the flow of patients from the OR to the PACU.

Because this problem relates to a population of patients, a team was assembled to conduct an evidence-based practice (EBP) project at an academic hospital. The EBP team consisted of 14 experienced PACU nurses representing three PACUs (two inpatient and one ambulatory outpatient). The nurses on the team included nurse clinicians at various levels, an educator, and a manager. These nurses were supported by School of Nursing faculty, a nurse researcher, and two nurse administrators experienced in standards of care and performance improvement.

The practice question posed was: For adult ambulatory surgery patients, does discharge from PACU prior to voiding versus discharge from PACU after voiding result in increased urinary retention?

Evidence

In an effort to resolve this dilemma, we reviewed the American Society of PeriAnesthesia Nurses (ASPAN) Standards, the professional nursing organization that guides this specialty practice. The standards did not directly address the issue nor were there any institutional guidelines to govern our practice. A literature search was conducted using CINAHL and PubMed. One hundred articles pertinent to voiding after surgery were identified. Fifty-nine articles were reviewed; 26 were applicable to the question.

Individual nurses were assigned specific article(s) to review and present to the group. A critique tool was used for each article based on the study's evidence type (experimental, quasi-experimental, guideline, systematic review, qualitative, performance improvement project, or financial analysis report). A PACU nurse and a mentor reviewed each article for consistency. Presenters of each article discussed the applicability, strength of evidence, lessons learned, and limitations of each article so the group could validate the presenter's rating.

Nine experimental studies, five quasi-experimental studies, three non-experimental studies, one guideline, and eight expert opinions were critiqued. ASPAN discharge standards were reviewed and the American Society of Anesthesia (ASA) was contacted. The ASA suggested that a patient's discharge prior to voiding should be evaluated on a case-by-case basis. Seventeen national teaching hospitals were contacted by telephone to determine their policy on discharging patients prior to voiding. Results indicated inconsistencies in policies and practice in discharging patients prior to voiding. Usually, a physician's order was needed to discharge the patient, but the criteria varied among physicians from different PACU Phase II settings (inpatient Phase II and ambulatory Phase II).

Subsequent recommendations were categorized in three levels (low risk, moderate risk, and high risk) for urinary retention based on patient history, anesthesia, or surgery. Low-risk ambulatory adult patients can be safely discharged prior to voiding. Although moderate-risk patients may be dischargeable with instructions to return within 6–8 hours if they have not voided, there was not enough evidence to make a recommendation. High-risk patients should void prior to discharge. A bladder scanner may be useful to identify urinary retention, but the group recognized the high cost of the scanner as a barrier in recommending its use.

Translation

The PACU team supported the policy change that low-risk patients can be safely discharged, and moderate and high-risk patients should void prior to discharge. The PACU discharge criteria were modified to reflect the EBP recommendations. PACU staff received education on the evidence and implications. Adult ambulatory patients who are discharged without voiding were given clear instructions to return to the hospital if urinary retention occurs. Voiding assessment was added to the next day patient phone follow-up. Since the guidelines were implemented, the PACU has not identified any problems with urinary retention or return to the emergency room related to bladder distention. Changes in length of stay or patient satisfaction were not measured.

In addition to an organizational impact on care, this project was used as an example to illustrate an evidence-based practice process for ASPAN as the society developed its evidence-based practice model.

2

Should Tube Feedings Be Held When Administering Phenytoin Suspension?

Sandra L. Dearholt, MS, RN
Barbara Fitzsimmons, MS, RN, CNRN
Brenda James-White, BSN, RN, CNRN
Susan Corn, BSN, RN, CNRN
Mary F. Boyle, BSN, RN, CNRN
Jane Adams, BSN, RN, CNRN
John Lewin, PharmD
Dawn Carlson, RD

Practice Question

Phenytoin (PHT) is considered the agent of choice for seizure prophylaxis, status epilepticus, and post-operative and post-trauma seizures. Current practice in the neuroscience department was to hold tube feedings (TF) for 2 hours before and 2 hours after administration of PHT suspension. This practice evolved due to concern regarding the potential for reducing seizure control because of the interaction of PHT and TF formulas. Even though the practice of holding TF was included as part of the hospital's food and drug interaction table in the medication administration policy, there was variation in practice across the hospital. In addition, the practice was time-consuming for the nursing staff and interfered with the patients' nutritional intake.

An interdisciplinary team, including nursing members of the neuroscience nursing standards of practice committee along with pharmacy and nutrition department staff, conducted an evidence-based practice (EBP) project to answer the following EBP question: Does the continuous infusion of enteral TF versus holding enteral TF for 2 hours before and 2 hours after the administration of PHT suspension have an effect on PHT levels in adult patients?

Evidence

To gather evidence, a literature search was conducted using CINAHL and PubMed. Five articles were reviewed. Included was one experimental study (Level I), one quasi-experimental study (Level II), one expert opinion based on evidence (Level IV), and two expert opinions (Level V). The quality of the Level I, II, and V evidence were rated as good (B), and the Level IV evidence quality was rated as high (A). The evidence revealed a long-standing controversy (first reported in 1982) surrounding the interaction between oral PHT and enteral TF, which is associated with a decrease in serum PHT concentrations. This mechanism is not fully explained. However, the results of the review identified no conclusive evidence that stopping TF 2 hours before and 2 hours after the administration of PHT suspension significantly increased serum PHT levels.

A search for national guidelines failed to produce any results. The practice question was then posted on the American Association of Neuroscience Nurses listserv. Four responses were obtained, identifying variation in practice. One hospital did not hold TF. The remaining three hospitals held TF for 1 hour before and 1 hour after.

Translation

Based on the appraisal of evidence, the EBP team made the recommendation to no longer hold TF 2 hours before and 2 hours after administration of PHT suspension and to continue close monitoring of PHT levels, including free PHT levels. This recommendation was made to the Pharmacy and Therapeutics (P&T) Committee, which is an interdisciplinary, hospital-level committee. The evidence was reviewed with key members of the committee. Because the EBP process was used and supporting evidence presented clearly, the physician chair of the P&T Committee approved the change in protocol without requiring the EBP team to present to the entire committee. This practice change has been in place for 1 year with no reported adverse events.

Pin Site Care

Susan Kulik, MSN, MBA, RN, ONC

Practice Question

During review of the skeletal pin site care protocol, surgical nurses on the Standards of Care Committee (SOC) noted that references supporting the protocol were outdated, frequency of pin site care was not addressed in the protocol, and use of hydrogen peroxide was recommended for wound care. In other hospital protocols, use of hydrogen peroxide had been discontinued as a routine agent for cleansing wounds because of concerns about slowing the healing process.

The pin care protocol guides nurses in the management of patients with an external fixator, a device used to treat a bone deformity or a fracture. This device is connected to the bone with screws commonly called *pins*, which are placed on either side of the fractured bone to hold the bone in place and to securely anchor the fixator. Infection at the pin insertion site is a common complication of external fixation; hence, ensuring the hospital protocol is consistent with evidence-based practices (EBP) is considered an important surgical nursing priority.

The EBP team was led by two nurse managers, one of whom sits on the hospital-wide SOC, and one with extensive experience conducting EBP projects. Each nursing unit in the department of surgery selected a nurse for the team, with representation from three intensive care units, two step-down units, eight inpatient units, two progressive care units, and the operating rooms. The team was supported by a nurse researcher, the director of surgical nursing, and the assistant director of surgical nursing. The chair of the department of orthopaedic surgery served as the physician liaison.

The practice question posed was: What is the most effective method in managing pin care among orthopaedic patients?

Evidence

The two team leaders searched the CINAHL and PubMed databases and gathered 15 articles on pin site care. Search terms used were: pin site, pin site care, skeletal pins, and external fixators. Team resource packets were developed to include EBP tools, prototype articles to practice critiquing with the tools, and the pin care articles needing review. A time line was developed that consisted of 3 meeting days, 4 hours at each session. The first meeting included an introduction of the participants, goals and objectives, and education on the Johns Hopkins Nursing Evidence-Based Practice model and guidelines (JHNEBP). Resource packets with EBP tools were distributed at this meeting. Team members were instructed to read the pin care articles as homework assignments for review and appraisal.

During the second meeting, the team reviewed the pin site care evidence and the completed individual evidence summations. An overall evidence summation, practice recommendations, and future plans were completed during the final meeting.

Although there were numerous published reports of pin site care protocols, research evidence regarding the effectiveness of these protocols was scant. Two experimental studies, two quasi-experimental studies, eight non-experimental studies, and three expert opinions were reviewed and critiqued. Two protocols from other teaching hospitals were obtained and reviewed. Two randomized controlled trials (RCT) and one quasi-experimental study were of good quality (B); most were of low quality (C), with no consistent or definitive results.

A multi-center RCT that randomized subjects to one of seven pin care protocols recommended cleansing with half-strength hydrogen peroxide and applying a Xeroform dressing to pin sites for best infection prevention. A second RCT revealed no differences between daily and weekly pin site care with chlorhexidene. Although these studies were of good quality, both recommended further research with larger sample sizes.

Both quasi-experimental studies recommended cleansing pin sites with chlorhexidene and one addressed frequency of pin care, but neither study demonstrated consistent results. Review of the three expert opinion articles revealed that clinicians make decisions about how to manage pin sites throughout their daily practices. Most of the experts recommended normal saline and a dry sterile dressing for pin site care. The use of chlorhexidene was advocated by the National Association of Orthopaedic Nurses (NAON), although this professional organization also recommended further research.

In summarizing the evidence reviewed in this project, there was no clear answer to how pin site care among orthopaedic patients should be conducted to reduce the potential for infection.

Translation

There is insufficient research evidence on which to base the management of pin site care. The evidence revealed inconsistency in the approach to managing pin site care among orthopaedic patients in preventing infection rates. There were no studies that examined the effectiveness of pin site care versus no care. Furthermore, it is not known if pin site care actually reduces infection rates.

The variation of research findings and the weak evidence found suggest there is insufficient evidence in recommending a single protocol for pin site care. The research evidence did appear consistent with the NAON guidelines for pin site care that were based on the experimental studies reviewed. These guidelines recommend the use of chlorhexidene for cleansing the pin site. The EBP team decided to adhere to these guidelines until further research supports a change in practice.

Support was secured from both physician and nursing leadership to implement changes in the existing pin site care protocol to change the agent for daily pin site cleansing from hydrogen peroxide to chlorhexidene. Nursing staff was educated about the evidence underlying this decision through poster presentations and staff meetings. The team plans to periodically review the literature for the appearance of new sources of evidence and to attend national conferences to maintain currency on the latest protocols. Additionally, the team is developing a research study on pin site care and is considering designing this as a multi-institutional study.

Summary

The examination of evidence on pin care management was a very valuable experience for team members. The EBP process increased awareness of the need to conduct further study on pin care management, because findings were not sufficient to support current practice. The pin care project stimulated the interest of participating nurses in doing other unit-based projects. These nurses have become unit-based EBP champions and are assisting their nursing colleagues in developing unit-based EBP questions. The project encouraged open discussion on how to make clinical changes and has increased the value in using EBP to support protocols.

4

Prevention of Post-Operative Urinary Retention After Uro-Gynecologic Surgery

Barbara L. Buchko, RN, MS
Leslie E. Robinson, MD
Paul H. Douglass, MD
John J. Lawrence, MD
Deb Fake, RN, ADN
Faye Hammers, RN, ADN
Jill Madigan, RNC, BSN

Practice Question

Urinary retention can be a significant post-operative problem for women undergoing uro-gynecologic surgery. Bladder distention can lead to impaired bladder function, urinary tract infections, and disruption of surgical repair with impaired surgical outcome. When a change in patient population led to an increased volume of uro-gynecologic surgery patients, nurses questioned the variation in physician practice. Both nurses and physicians were concerned when a few of the patients had bladder distention with subsequent catheterizations for 800 and 1000 cc of urine, and one patient's surgical site needed repair. Both physicians and nurses identified the need for:

- a definition of urinary retention, as physician orders varied

- enhanced nursing skill and knowledge of the bladder scanner

- prescribed indications for catheterization of the patient

- consistent documentation of voiding trial results.

The practice question agreed upon by this interdisciplinary team was: What is the best way to prevent urinary retention and bladder distention following gynecologic and uro-gynecologic procedures?

Evidence

Thirty-two sources of evidence from CINAHL and PubMed were reviewed using the Johns Hopkins Nursing Evidence-Based Practice model (JHNEBP). Of 32 sources of evidence reviewed, five were excluded. Of the remaining 27, none was experimental, two were quasi-experimental, 18 were non-experimental or qualitative, seven were integrative or systematic reviews, and none was expert opinion or guidelines.

In the prevention of urinary retention and subsequent bladder distention, the strongest evidence (Level II) supported the following summary:

- High-risk patients should be observed and assessed until bladder is emptied to avoid urinary retention. High-risk was defined as: history of voiding problems (assess prior to surgery)

  - Older (over 50 years of age)

  - Spinal anesthesia

  - Type of surgery (hernia and anal)

  - Volume of IV fluids operatively > 1000 ml

  - Use of narcotics for post-operative pain control

- Bladder ultrasound (US) is a viable option to prevent urinary retention

Level III evidence supporting the summary includes:

- Identify post-operative urinary retention (POUR) in the post-anesthesia recovery unit with a bladder scanner

- Voiding efficiency should be > 50%

- Primary retention > 500 ml can lead to further catheterization, > 1000 ml can lead to further hospitalization

- Documentation of management of POUR is critical

- Normal bladder capacity 400–600 ml

- First urge to void 150–300 ml

- Over-distended bladder generally defined as 500–1000 ml

This evidence needs to be considered in the prevention of post-operative urinary retention and bladder distention.

Translation

Based on the evidence, the interdisciplinary team created an algorithm that defined urinary retention, post-void residual, voiding efficiency, when and how to assess the patient, when to catheterize (either intermittent or continuous), and success (or when measurement could be discontinued). The algorithm was designed using clinical judgment (abdominal palpation) and ultrasound techniques (bladder scanner) to evaluate post voiding residual and voiding efficiency.

Clinical nurses were educated on the use of the algorithm as well as physiology of the urinary tract, normal voiding function, post-operative voiding complications, techniques to monitor and diagnose malfunction of voiding process, how to measure for post-void residual, the concept of voiding efficiency, and use of ultrasound technology for monitoring voiding function. The nurses on the team also observed return demonstrations with use of the bladder scanner.

A non-experimental comparative design was used to evaluate patient outcomes before and after education and algorithm implementation. The institutional review board at the hospital approved the project. Data were extracted by retrospective chart review comparing women cared for post uro-gynecologic surgery prior to the development of the algorithm and after the initiation of the algorithm and subsequent nursing education. The following information was included on the data abstraction tool:

- Date and time of continuous catheter insertion (determined by 15 minutes prior to time of incision)

- Date and time of continuous catheter removal (determined by either documented actual time or time of completion of surgery)

- Date, time, and amount of voiding

- Time and amount of post-void residual measured by either bladder scanner or intermittent catheterization after each void.

Overall, 56 medical records were reviewed. Twelve patients had re-insertion of a continuous catheter. Therefore, there were 68 voiding trials initiated with 312 bladder assessments. In the "before" group, there were 21 patients representing 27 voiding trials and 195 bladder assessments and 29% of the continuous catheter re-insertions. In the "after" group, there were 35 patients representing 47 voiding trials and 117 bladder assessments representing 17% of the continuous catheter re-insertions.

Utilizing chi-square analysis to determine if patients were catheterized when there was greater than 300 ml of urine in the bladder demonstrated a p value of .096 (before group 58% and after group 67%). Based on this finding, the team surmised that the potential for damage to the surgical site would decrease because of the increase in the assessment and recognition of urinary retention. The frequency of intermittent catheterization was analyzed also using chi-square analysis. There was no significance with a p value of 0.2, however, a trend toward decreased frequency was noted with the before group at 43% and the after group at 26%. There was almost no difference in the length of time of continuous catheterization between the groups.

Summary

This project has positively impacted patient care in many ways. First, it created sensitivity to current post-operative practice in the management of post-operative urinary retention and bladder distention for the obstetrical and gynecologic patient. Second, it identified the necessity of education for nurses concerning post-operative urinary retention and bladder distention. Only 56 percent of the nurses attended the education offered. If all the nurses had participated in the education, it is possible there would have been significant improvement in patient outcomes. Last, more thorough documentation is improving communication between nurses and physicians; however, inconsistencies in documentation remain an issue.

Next Steps

1. Implement mandatory computer-based training using case studies and questions focused on understanding bladder capacity and urinary retention, with bladder distention and nursing actions to be implemented.

2. Create a standardized order set to replace the algorithm.

3. Computerized documentation for consistency of documentation with computerized calculation of the voiding efficiency.

4. Standardization for care is being disseminated to general surgical units as gynecologic patients may be cared for on another general surgical unit when necessary. The hospital-wide nursing practice council (NPC) has been approached with a request for acceptance of the standard orders throughout the hospital. In addition, the team has requested recommendations from the NPC on how to provide this education to all staff nurses. These requests were met with acceptance and encouragement, as the information was based on evidence.

5. The NPC has requested changes to the standard of care of all post-operative patients to include the evidence for prevention and management of post-operative urinary retention, so that best outcomes can be obtained by all.

5

Nursing Strategies to Decrease Patient Physical and Verbal Violence

Judy Meyers, MSN, RN

Kathleen M. White, PhD, RN, CNAA, BC

Practice Question

After the completion of several evidence-based practice (EBP) projects at The Johns Hopkins Hospital, the Johns Hopkins Nursing Evidence-Based Practice (JHNEBP) team sought to test the JHNEBP model in other types of facilities. The director of a small, rural state hospital on the eastern shore of Maryland had expressed interest in having the model and guidelines presented to her staff. This interest presented an opportunity for both parties.

Two conference calls were held with the director of nursing, Judy Meyers, and her clinical leaders to plan the implementation. Meyers completed an organizational assessment of her facility. Information was gathered about the facility's resources, including access to databases, journals, availability of audio-visual equipment, and workshop support. The last call centered on the development of a narrowly defined practice question of interest to the facility and a plan to take the 2-day training method used in the model testing to complete an EBP project at that facility.

At the conclusion of the call, the practice question was identified as:

> For patients assessed with a propensity for a violent episode, what nursing strategies should be implemented to decrease the likelihood of violence?

Evidence

The EBP team members conducted a literature search using the online CINAHL database with the key words "assessment for violence" and "strategies to decrease violence." The evidence was gathered and sent to the rural hospital with instructions to distribute the material to the future project participants along with the evidence appraisal tools.

All the EBP training was conducted on-site at the rural hospital. The first day of the program introduced EBP using the JHNEBP model and guidelines, including the Practice question, Evidence, and Translation (PET) process; the necessary tools for EBP; and how to conduct an evidence search. Day 2 was focused on developing skills for appraising the strength and quality of the evidence, identifying gaps, and summarizing the evidence to make recommendations for next steps.

Seventeen sources of evidence were reviewed, including one quasi-experimental study, seven non-experimental studies, one qualitative study, one quality improvement study, one case study evaluation, and four expert opinion articles. The evidence supported the need for assessment and proactive prevention of violent episodes.

Based on this evidence, the group made several recommendations:

1. Staff nurses must be educated about parameters for violence assessment and the preventive/proactive interventions that are possible.

2. Clinical leadership team members should review the components of their current training program, such as the timing, frequency, modes of training, delivery, and components to be researched.

3. Clinical leadership team members should consider developing an algorithm to support their decision making.

4. Administrative support for debriefing after a violent episode should be provided, and the leadership team should require that debriefing data be given to the staff by nursing quality improvement, so the nurses can learn from the events and better respond in the future.

5. Preventive/proactive violence interventions should be included in performance data collection.

6. Assessment tools for violence should be reviewed on an ongoing basis.

Translation

Since the completion of the project, the hospital nursing group has used the outcomes of the project in preparation for its Joint Commission visit. The group used the evidence to develop a violence risk assessment tool (see Figure 10.1) and guidelines for implementing interventions based on the patient's risk score of low, moderate, or high risk for violence (see Figure 10.2). They developed a pilot study for fiscal year 2006 on two of their inpatient units to complete the assessment on all newly admitted patients (see Figure 10.3). They have had a decrease in staff assaults by patients and increased communication among staff members through their group work.

Summary

This project surpassed expectations. The EBP team was extremely pleased with the participation and enthusiasm on the part of the nursing clinical leadership at the rural hospital. The rural hospital staff found the EBP process practical and easy to use in its facility.

Violence Risk Assessment

Completed By: _____   Date: _____

Gender   Male [   ]   Female [   ]

Date of Last Violence Risk Assessment and Score _____

Long-term behavior	**YES**	**NO**
1. Does the patient have history of violence directed toward self or others?	____	____
If the answer to 1. is "yes," was this violence associated with substance abuse?	____	____

Risk factors

2. Active paranoid delusions	____	____
3. Hallucinations associated with negative affect	____	____
4. Manic state	____	____
5. Neurological abnormalities	____	____
6. Alcohol or drug intoxication and withdrawal states	____	____

Immediate Situation

7. Is there forensic involvement or PC commitment?	____	____
8. Is the patient verbally or non-verbally threatening staff or peers?	____	____

TOTAL SCORE [   ]

LOW RISK = Zero (0) to two (2) Yes answers
MODERATE RISK = Three (3) to Five (5) Yes answers
HIGH RISK = Six (6) and above

Figure 10.1. Violence Risk Assessment

LOW RISK

- Search patient and patient's immediate environment for harmful objects.

- Assess privilege level if applicable.

- Review the De-Escalation Tab in E-Chart (Patient's Interdisciplinary Assessment).

- Assess patient's dorm assignment. May want to move closer to the nurse station or to the mini-ward. The mini-ward is an unlocked, self-contained suite located adjacent to the nursing station. It is composed of a central hallway and a sitting room—both visible from one side of the nursing station or by video monitoring—and bathrooms. All newly admitted patients are assigned to a private room in the mini-ward until admission assessments are completed by all departments. In addition, any patient who may need to be temporarily housed away from other patients on the unit, for reasons other than infection control, may be temporarily assigned to the mini-ward.

- Place in anger management group.

- Educate regarding consequences of actions (Hospital philosophy for zero tolerance of violence).

- Assess every 30 minutes, offer prn medication as needed, utilize interventions noted in De-Escalation Tab, and assess effectiveness.

MODERATE RISK

- Search patient and patient's immediate environment for harmful objects.

- Assess privilege level and possibly place the patient on assault, suicide, or fire setting advisory.

- Review the De-Escalation Tab in E-Chart (Patient's Interdisciplinary Assessment).

- Determine, if possible, patient's intent by asking probing questions:

  - Are you angry at anyone? If yes, who?
  - Are you thinking about hurting anyone?
  - If yes, when and where?
  - Do you have a plan?
  - Is the patient able to verbally interact with staff and provide assurance that he or she will be able to refrain from any actions that may be harmful to himself or herself or others?

  o Tell the patient to let staff know if "you are unable to control your behavior."

- Assess patient's dorm assignment. May want to move closer to the nurse station or to the mini-ward.

- Place in anger management group.

- Educate regarding consequences of actions (Hospital philosophy for zero tolerance of violence).

- Assess for elopement risk.

- If advisory status is implemented, assess every 15 minutes, offer prn medication as needed, utilize interventions noted in De-Escalation Tab, and assess effectiveness

HIGH RISK

- Search patient and patient's immediate environment for harmful objects.

- Assess patient's dorm assignment. Move closer to the nurse station or in back mini-ward.

- Assess privilege level and possibly place the patient on assault, suicide, elopement, or fire setting precautions.

- Determine patient's possible intent by asking probing questions:

  - Are you angry at anyone? If yes, who?

  - Are you thinking about hurting anyone? If yes, when and where?

  - Do you have a plan?

  - Is the patient able to verbally interact with staff and provide assurance that he or she will be able to refrain from any actions that may be harmful to himself or herself or others?

  - Tell the patient to let staff know if "you are unable to control your behavior."

- Assess for elopement risk. Notify hospital police if patient is placed on precautions.

- If precaution status is implemented, assess continuously, offer prn medication as needed, use interventions noted in De-Escalation Tab, and assess effectiveness.

Figure 10.2. Guidelines for Use of Violence Risk Assessment

Violence Risk Assessment

Pilot Plan, Fiscal Year 2006
Nanticoke & Choptank Units

Guidelines for Use

1. The clinical nurse specialist will complete on all newly admitted patients. (Note: Scores have already been obtained for the current patient population.)

2. Assessment score(s) will be shared with unit staff and the patient's treatment team.

3. Any or all of the interventions may be implemented by the treatment team based on the patient's total score.

4. Re-assessments are to be done by the clinical nurse specialist for the following:

   a. Change in patient's behavior.

   b. Evaluation for privileges (request for treatment mall privileges). Share score with the patient's treatment team and the forensic review board if applicable.

   c. Transfer from Nanticoke Unit to Choptank Unit.

5. The clinical nurse specialist will retain the scoring forms to allow for possible retrospective review.

Tool validity was conducted by a preliminary review on data gathered in July 2005 on all patients on the Nanticoke & Choptank units.

- Modification of the assessment tool occurred.

- Several questions addressed the patient's past history of violence. These were consolidated, and the number of questions dropped from 10 to 8.

The interventions were modified to include the De-Escalation Tab noted in the new E-Chart Record and to assess for elopement potential when the patient's score places him / her in the high-risk category. Notification to hospital police when the patient's score falls in the high-risk category.

Inter-rater reliability will be conducted at the 3-month interval. The CNS from Nanticoke will do random assessments on (5) five Choptank patients and the Choptank CNS will do random ratings on (5) Nanticoke patients. Comparison of the scores will be conducted.

Reevaluation of this pilot will occur in 6 months.

Figure 10.3.   Violence Risk Assessment Pilot Plan for Fiscal Year 2006

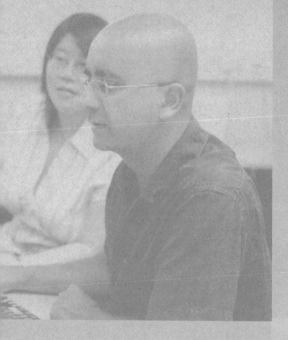

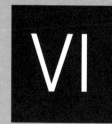

VI

Appendixes

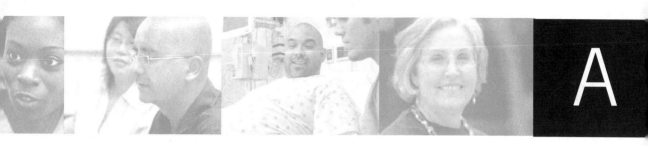

Question Development Tool

Question Development Tool

What is the practice issue?

1. **What is the practice area?**	☐ Clinical	☐ Education	☐ Administration

2. How was the practice issue identified? (Check all that apply)

- ☐ Safety/risk management concerns
- ☐ Unsatisfactory patient outcomes
- ☐ Wide variations in practice
- ☐ Significant financial concerns
- ☐ Difference between hospital and community practice
- ☐ Clinical practice issue is a concern
- ☐ Procedure or process is a time waster
- ☐ Clinical practice issue has no scientific base

3. **What is the scope of the problem?**	☐ Individual ☐ Population ☐ Institution/system

4. What are the PICO Components?

P – (Patient, Population, or Problem):

I – (Intervention):

C – (Comparison with other treatments, if applicable):

O – (Outcomes):

5. What evidence must be gathered? (Check all that apply)

- ☐ Literature Search
- ☐ Standards (Regulatory, Professional, Community)
- ☐ Guidelines
- ☐ Expert Opinion
- ☐ Patient Preferences
- ☐ Clinical Expertise
- ☐ Financial Analysis

6. State the search question in narrow, manageable terms:

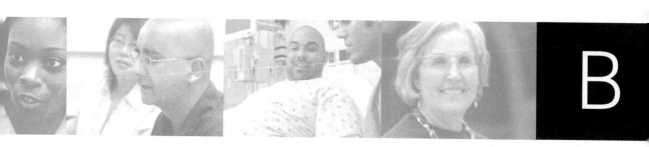

B

Evidence Rating Scale

Evidence Rating Scale

STRENGTH of the Evidence	
Level I	Experimental study/randomized controlled trial (RCT) or meta analysis of RCT
Level II	Quasi-experimental study
Level III	Non-experimental study, qualitative study, or meta-synthesis.
Level IV	Opinion of nationally recognized experts based on research evidence or expert consensus panel (systematic review, clinical practice guidelines)
Level V	Opinion of individual expert based on non-research evidence. (Includes case studies; literature review; organizational experience e.g., quality improvement and financial data; clinical expertise, or personal experience)

QUALITY of the Evidence		
A	High	Research	consistent results with sufficient sample size, adequate control, and definitive conclusions; consistent recommendations based on extensive literature review that includes thoughtful reference to scientific evidence.
		Summative reviews	well-defined, reproducible search strategies; consistent results with sufficient numbers of well defined studies; criteria-based evaluation of overall scientific strength and quality of included studies; definitive conclusions.
		Organizational	well-defined methods using a rigorous approach; consistent results with sufficient sample size; use of reliable **and** valid measures
		Expert Opinion	expertise is clearly evident
B	Good	Research	reasonably consistent results, sufficient sample size, some control, with fairly definitive conclusions; reasonably consistent recommendations based on fairly comprehensive literature review that includes some reference to scientific evidence
		Summative reviews	reasonably thorough and appropriate search; reasonably consistent results with sufficient numbers of well defined studies; evaluation of strengths and limitations of included studies; fairly definitive conclusions.
		Organizational	Well-defined methods; reasonably consistent results with sufficient numbers; use of **reliable and valid** measures; reasonably consistent recommendations
		Expert Opinion	expertise appears to be credible.
C	Low quality or major flaws	Research	little evidence with inconsistent results, insufficient sample size, conclusions cannot be drawn
		Summative reviews	undefined, poorly defined, or limited search strategies; insufficient evidence with inconsistent results; conclusions cannot be drawn
		Organizational	Undefined, **or** poorly defined methods; insufficient sample size; inconsistent results; undefined, poorly defined or measures that lack adequate reliability or validity
		Expert Opinion	expertise is not discernable or is dubious.

*A study rated an A would be of high quality, whereas a study rated a C would have major flaws that raise serious questions about the believability of the findings and should be automatically eliminated from consideration.

Newhouse R, Dearholt S, Poe S, Pugh LC, & White K. (2007). The Johns Hopkins Nursing Evidence-Based Practice Rating Scale. Baltimore, MD: The Johns Hopkins Hospital, Johns Hopkins University School of Nursing.

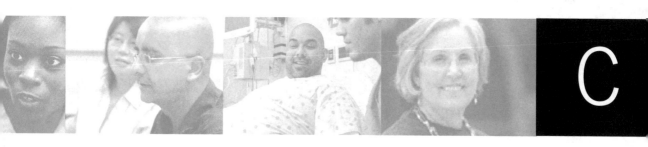

Johns Hopkins
Nursing Evidence-Based
Practice Model

Johns Hopkins Nursing Evidence-Based Practice Model

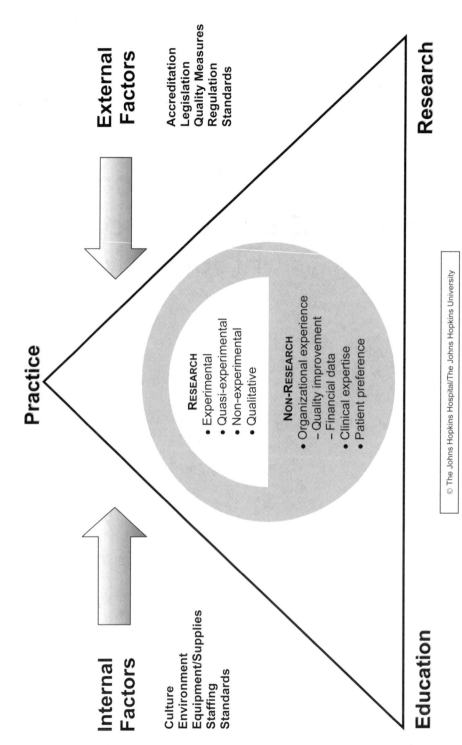

External Factors

Accreditation
Legislation
Quality Measures
Regulation
Standards

Practice

Research

RESEARCH
- Experimental
- Quasi-experimental
- Non-experimental
- Qualitative

NON-RESEARCH
- Organizational experience
  – Quality improvement
  – Financial data
- Clinical expertise
- Patient preference

Internal Factors

Culture
Environment
Equipment/Supplies
Staffing
Standards

Education

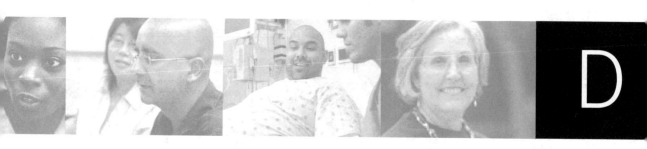

D

Practice Question,
Evidence, Translation
(PET)

The Johns Hopkins Nursing Evidence-Based Practice Process

PET (Practice Question, Evidence, and Translation)

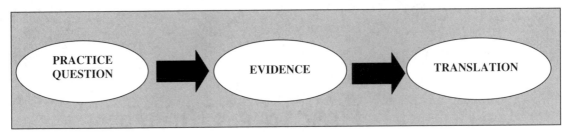

PRACTICE QUESTION

STEP 1: Identify an EBP question
STEP 2: Define the scope of the practice question
STEP 3: Assign responsibility for leadership
STEP 4: Recruit an interdisciplinary team
STEP 5: Schedule a team conference

EVIDENCE

STEP 6: Conduct an internal and external search for evidence
STEP 7: Appraise all types of evidence
STEP 8: Summarize the evidence
STEP 9: Rate the strength of the evidence
STEP 10: Develop recommendations for change in systems or processes of care based on the strength of the evidence

TRANSLATION

STEP 11: Determine the appropriateness and feasibility of translating recommendations into the specific practice setting
STEP 12: Create an action plan
STEP 13: Implement the change
STEP 14: Evaluate outcomes
STEP 15: Report the results of the preliminary evaluation to decision makers
STEP 16: Secure support from decision makers to implement the recommended change internally
STEP 17: Identify the next steps
STEP 18: Communicate the findings

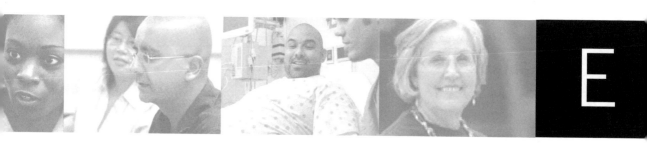

Project Management

Project Management

Practice Question:

EBP Team Leader(s):

EBP Team Members:

Overall Aim:

	Start Date	Days Required	End Date	Person Assigned	Milestone	Comment / Resources Required
PRACTICE QUESTION:						
Step 1: Identify an EBP question						
Step 2: Define the scope of the practice question						
Step 3: Assign responsibility for leadership						
Step 4: Recruit an interdisciplinary team						
Step 5: Schedule a team conference						
EVIDENCE:						
Step 6: Conduct an internal and external search for evidence						
Step 7: Appraise all types of evidence						
Step 8: Summarize the evidence						
Step 9: Rate the strength of the evidence						
Step 10: Develop recommendations for change in systems or processes of care based on the strength of the evidence						
TRANSLATION:						
Step 11: Determine the appropriateness and feasibility of translating recommendations into the specific practice setting						
Step 12: Create an action plan						
Step 13: Implement the change						
Step 14: Evaluate outcomes						
Step 15: Report the results of preliminary evaluation to decision makers						
Step 16: Secure support from decision makers to implement the recommended change internally						
Step 17: Identify the next steps						
Step 18: Communicate the findings						

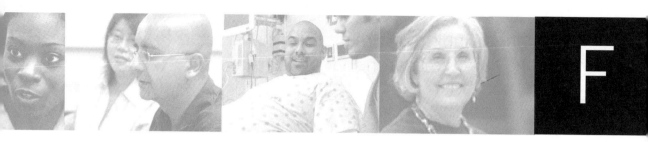

Johns Hopkins Nursing
Evidence-Based Practice
Research Evidence Appraisal

Johns Hopkins Nursing Evidence-Based Practice Research Evidence Appraisal

Evidence Level: _____

ARTICLE TITLE:		NUMBER:
AUTHOR(S):		DATE:
JOURNAL:		
SETTING:	SAMPLE (COMPOSITION/SIZE)	

☐ Experimental	☐ Meta-analysis	☐ Quasi-experimental	☐ Non-experimental	☐ Qualitative	☐ Meta-synthesis

Does this study apply to the population targeted by my practice question?	☐Yes	☐No

If the answer is No, STOP here (unless there are similar characteristics).

Strength of Study Design

	Yes	No
• Was sample size adequate and appropriate?	☐Yes	☐No
• Were study participants randomized?	☐Yes	☐No
• Was there an intervention?	☐Yes	☐No
• Was there a control group?	☐Yes	☐No
• If there was more than one group, were groups equally treated, except for the intervention?	☐Yes	☐No
• Was there adequate description of the data collection methods?	☐Yes	☐No

Study Results

	Yes	No
• Were results clearly presented?	☐Yes	☐No
• Was an interpretation/analysis provided?	☐Yes	☐No

Study Conclusions

	Yes	No
• Were conclusions based on clearly presented results?	☐Yes	☐No
• Were study limitations identified and discussed?	☐Yes	☐No

PERTINENT STUDY FINDINGS AND RECOMMENDATIONS

Will the results help in caring for my patients?	☐Yes	☐No

Evidence Rating (scales on back)

Strength of Evidence	
Quality of Evidence (check one)	☐ High (A) ☐ Good (B) ☐ Low/Major flaw (C)

Johns Hopkins Nursing Evidence-Based Practice Research Evidence Appraisal

Strength of Evidence
Level I (Strong)

EXPERIMENTAL STUDY (RANDOMIZED CONTROLLED TRIAL OR RCT)
- Study participants (subjects) are randomly assigned to either a treatment (TX) or control (non-treatment) group
- May be:
  o Blind: subject does not know which TX subject is receiving
  o Double-blind: neither subject nor investigator knows which TX subject is receiving
  o Non-blind: both subject and investigator know which TX subject is receiving; used when it is felt that the knowledge of treatment is unimportant

META-ANALYSIS OF RCTs
- Quantitatively synthesizes and analyzes results of multiple primary studies addressing a similar research question
- Statistically pools results from independent but combinable studies
- Summary statistic (effect size) is expressed in terms of direction (positive, negative, or zero) and magnitude (high, medium, small)

Level II

QUASI-EXPERIMENTAL STUDY
- Always includes manipulation of an independent variable
- Lacks either random assignment or control group
- Findings must be considered in light of threats to validity (particularly selection)

Level III

NON-EXPERIMENTAL STUDY
- No manipulation of the independent variable
- Can be descriptive, comparative, or relational
- Often uses secondary data
- Findings must be considered in light of threats to validity (particularly selection, lack of severity or co-morbidity adjustment)

QUALITATIVE STUDY
- Explorative in nature, such as interviews, observations, or focus groups
- Starting point for studies of questions for which little research currently exists
- Sample sizes are usually small and study results are used to design stronger studies that are more objective and quantifiable

META-SYNTHESIS
- Research technique that critically analyzes and synthesizes findings from qualitative research
- Identifies key concepts and metaphors and determines their relationships to each other
- Aim is not to produce a summary statistic, but rather to interpret and translate findings

Quality of Evidence (Scientific Evidence)

A High: consistent results, sufficient sample size, adequate control, and definitive conclusions; consistent recommendations based on extensive literature review that includes thoughtful reference to scientific evidence

B Good: reasonably consistent results, sufficient sample size, some control, and fairly definitive conclusions; reasonably consistent recommendations based on fairly comprehensive literature review that includes some reference to scientific evidence

C Low/Major flaw: little evidence with inconsistent results, insufficient sample size, conclusions cannot be drawn

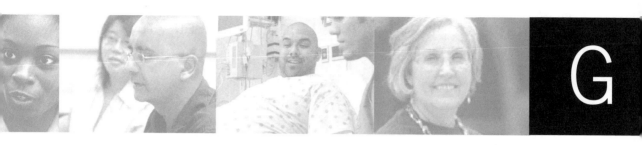

Johns Hopkins Nursing
Evidence-Based Practice
Non-Research
Evidence Appraisal

Johns Hopkins Nursing Evidence-Based Practice Non-Research Evidence Appraisal

Evidence Level: _____

ARTICLE TITLE:	NUMBER:
AUTHOR(S):	DATE:
JOURNAL:	

☐ Systematic Review	☐ Clinical Practice Guidelines	☐ Organizational (QI, financial data)	☐ Expert opinion, case study, literature review

Does evidence apply to the population targeted by my practice question?	☐ Yes	☐ No
If the answer is No, STOP here (unless there are similar characteristics).		

Systematic Review

• Is the question clear?	☐ Yes	☐ No
• Was a rigorous peer-reviewed process used?	☐ Yes	☐ No
• Are search strategies specified, and reproducible?	☐ Yes	☐ No
• Are search strategies appropriate to include all pertinent studies?	☐ Yes	☐ No
• Are criteria for inclusion and exclusion of studies specified?	☐ Yes	☐ No
• Are details of included studies (design, methods, analysis) presented?	☐ Yes	☐ No
• Are methodological limitations disclosed?	☐ Yes	☐ No
• Are the variables in the studies reviewed similar, so that studies can be combined?	☐ Yes	☐ No

Clinical Practice Guidelines

• Were appropriate stakeholders involved in the development of this guideline?	☐ Yes	☐ No
• Are groups to which guidelines apply and do not apply clearly stated?	☐ Yes	☐ No
• Have potential biases been eliminated?	☐ Yes	☐ No
• Were guidelines valid (reproducible search, expert consensus, independent review, current, and level of supporting evidence identified for each recommendation)?	☐ Yes	☐ No
• Are recommendations clear?	☐ Yes	☐ No

Organizational Experience

• Was the aim of the project clearly stated?	☐ Yes	☐ No
• Is the setting similar to setting of interest?	☐ Yes	☐ No
• Was the method adequately described?	☐ Yes	☐ No
• Were measures identified?	☐ Yes	☐ No
• Were results adequately described?	☐ Yes	☐ No
• Was interpretation clear and appropriate?	☐ Yes	☐ No

Individual expert opinion, case study, literature review

• Was evidence based on the opinion of an individual?	☐ Yes	☐ No
• Is the individual an expert on the topic?	☐ Yes	☐ No
• Is author's opinion based on scientific evidence?	☐ Yes	☐ No
• Is the author's opinion clearly stated?	☐ Yes	☐ No
• Are potential biases acknowledged?	☐ Yes	☐ No

PERTINENT CONCLUSIONS AND RECOMMENDATIONS

Were conclusions based on the evidence presented?	☐ Yes	☐ No
Will the results help me in caring for my patients?	☐ Yes	☐ No

Quality of Evidence (scale on back):

Basic quality rating of the study under review (check one)	☐ High (A)	☐ Good (B)	☐ Low/Major flaw (C)

Johns Hopkins Nursing Evidence-Based Practice Non-Research Evidence Appraisal

Strength of Evidence
Level I-IV

SYSTEMATIC REVIEW
- Research review that compiles and summarizes evidence from research studies related to a specific clinical question
- Employs comprehensive search strategies and rigorous appraisal methods
- Contains an evaluation of strengths and limitations of studies under review
- If peer-reviewed process such as Cochrane is used, rate at the level of the research evidence included in the review if not a meta-analysis, which is rated at level I. If non-peer reviewed, rate at Level IV

Level IV

CLINICAL PRACTICE GUIDELINES
- Research and experiential evidence review that systematically develops statements that are meant to guide decision-making for specific clinical circumstances
- Evidence is appraised and synthesized from three basic sources: scientific findings, clinician expertise, and patient preferences

Level V (Weak)

ORGANIZATIONAL
- Review of quality improvement studies and financial analysis reports
- Evidence is appraised and synthesized from two basic sources: internal reports and external published reports

EXPERT OPINION, CASE STUDY, LITERATURE REVIEW
- Opinion of a nationally recognized expert based on non-research evidence (includes case studies, literature review, or personal experience)

Quality of Evidence (Summative Reviews)

A High: well-defined, reproducible search strategies; consistent results with sufficient numbers of well-designed studies; criteria-based evaluation of overall scientific strength and quality of included studies, and definitive conclusions

B Good: reasonably thorough and appropriate search; reasonably consistent results, sufficient numbers of well-designed studies, evaluation of strengths and limitations of included studies, with fairly definitive results

C Low/Major flaw: undefined, poorly defined, or limited search strategies; insufficient evidence with inconsistent results, conclusions cannot be drawn

Quality of Evidence (Expert Opinion)

A High: expertise is clearly evident

B Good: expertise appears to be credible

C Low/Major flaw: expertise is not discernable or is dubious

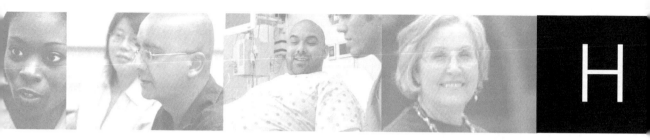

Individual Evidence Summary

Individual Evidence Summary

EBP Question _____

Date _____

#	Author	Date	Evidence Type	Sample & Sample Size	Results/ Recommendations	Limitations	RATING Strength/ Quality
				□ N/A			/
				□ N/A			/
				□ N/A			/
				□ N/A			/
				□ N/A			/
				□ N/A			/
				□ N/A			/
				□ N/A			/
				□ N/A			/
				□ N/A			/
				□ N/A			/
				□ N/A			/

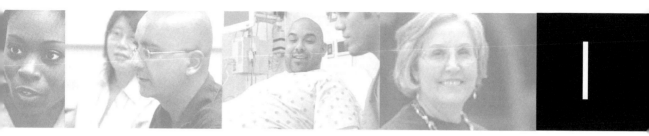

Overall Evidence
Summation

Overall Evidence Summation

Current Practice:

Evidence-Based Practice Question:

Level of Evidential Strength	Number of Studies	Summary of Findings	Overall Quality
I Experimental (randomized controlled trial – RCT) or meta-analysis of RCTs			
II Quasi-experimental			
III Non-experimental or qualitative			
IV Opinion of nationally recognized experts based on research evidence			
V Opinion of individual expert based on non-research evidence			

RECOMMENDATION(S):

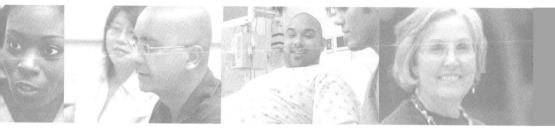

Index

D

E